Read All About It

Q's & A's About Nutrition, Volume II

To Karen – Enjoy – [signature] 2018

Dr. Phylis B. Canion

authorHOUSE®

AuthorHouse™
1663 Liberty Drive
Bloomington, IN 47403
www.authorhouse.com
Phone: 1-800-839-8640

First published by AuthorHouse   6/8/2011

ISBN: 978-1-4567-6783-9 (sc)
ISBN: 978-1-4567-6782-2 (hc)
ISBN: 978-1-4567-6781-5 (e)

Library of Congress Control Number: 2011908384

Printed in the United States of America

**To all that believe nutrition
is the secret to good health**

Q:

I am a cancer survivor and see lists from time to time of what foods I need to avoid, but very seldom do I see a list of what foods are recommended. Do you have a "top ten" list of the best of the best that a cancer survivor should eat?

A:

The National Cancer Institute estimates that roughly one-third of all cancer deaths may be diet related. Many of the common foods we eat contain cancer fighting properties from antioxidants to phytochemicals rather than the genetically modified processed foods. While there isn't a single element in a particular food that does all of the work, eating a variety of the best foods can help immensely. Here are some recommendations; Avocados are rich in glutathione, cruciferous vegetables like broccoli, cabbage, kale, Brussels sprouts and cauliflower have a chemical component called indole-3-carbinol that have the ability to convert cancer promoting estrogen into a more protective variety. Cruciferous vegetables also contain two important antioxidants, leutin and zeaxanthin that can play an important role in the diet of individuals with prostate cancer. Flax, which contains lignans is also high in omega-3 fatty acids, and garlic which has immune enhancing allium compounds. Certain mushrooms like shiitake, maitake, reishi, and coriolus versicolor can stimulate the production of interferon in the body as many studies have indicated in Japan. Nuts contain quercetin, while lemons, oranges, papayas and raspberries contain limonene, vitamin c and anthocyanins that are all antioxidants. Sweet potatoes and carrots contain beta-carotene and my all-time favorite and very popular in South America is tapioca, which is derived from the cassava plant and is very rich in nutrients. Decaffeinated green tea contains polyphenols which can be a relaxing benefit to the system. A few other tips; do not over cook your food, avoid the microwave, drink plenty of alkaline water, chew your food at least fifteen to twenty times before swallowing, avoid caffeine, get a good night's sleep and take your vitamins every day which can help build your immune system! Cancer is a disease of the body, mind and spirit. A proactive and positive spirit will help the cancer warrior be a survivor.

Q:

What are the most important toxins to avoid during pregnancy that may contaminate my food and water?

A:

While it would be nearly impossible to avoid exposure to all toxic chemicals, there are chemicals that can be easily avoided during pregnancy to protect the mother and baby. The worst chemicals with the most common exposure that awareness can help eliminate are Perfluorooctanate or PFOA's, Perfluorooctane Sulfonate, or PFOS's, Phthalates and Bisphenol A, more commonly referred to BPA. PFOA's and PFOS's exposure can be eliminated by avoiding the use of non-stick cookware, microwave popcorn bags, packaging for greasy foods in the food line and further exposure can be prevented by avoiding the use of stain proof clothing, carpet and fabric protectors and flame retardants. Phthalates are commonly found in hairsprays, cosmetics, perfumes, shampoos, conditioners, lotions and hair growth stimulators.(Phthalates are also in plastic toys that children chew on). BPA's are commonly found in plastic containers such as water bottles, sippy cups, pacifiers, plastic gallon milk bottles, and food and drink cans that have a plastic liner on the inside. As I always recommend, it is important to read the label on any product that you purchase, regardless if it is a food/ consumable product, clothing or toy and look for the above PFOA, PFOS, or BPA to be listed in the laundry list of ingredients. Also, look at the bottom of any plastic product to check out the number in the recycle triangle and avoid it if the number is a three, six or seven!

Q:

Can you share with me any secrets on cooking venison and wild game? My wife would appreciate it very much!

A:

Water is your best friend when cooking game meats. Venison tends to dry out quickly since it contains less fat and should never be overcooked. The flavor of wild game can be improved by soaking the meat in a solution of one half water and one half vinegar for one hour before cooking. This acts like a marinade and a tenderizer. To make juicy game burgers, simply add one third cup of cold water per pound of meat before mixing and grilling. For your meatloaf, just rub a small amount of water on top. And the suggestion you are waiting for, and your wife will appreciate the most, use a small can of ginger ale to cook your wild game in to eliminate that gamy flavor!

Q:

I am positioning myself to begin a weight loss program after the first of the year and have read some articles on the benefits of Leptin and weight loss. Can you explain?

A:

Your appetite is controlled by hormones. Jeffrey Friedman, M.D., a professor at Rockefeller University, discovered a hormone called leptin, that sends a crucial signal to your brain that allows you to control your eating. According to Robert J. Rowen, M.D., your fat cells make leptin in proportion to the amount of energy they have stored. Therefore, if your cells have plenty of calories in reserve, the cells will produce leptin to send the signal you are full. When the system is working properly, leptin turns off your appetite. However, when the system is out of balance, the lack of leptin will cause the exact opposite- a voracious appetite. To explain a bit further, there are two different types of cells in the hypothalamus, a region of the brain directly connected to the pituitary, where one cell stimulates your appetite while the other suppresses your appetite. It is the job of leptin to activate the appetite suppressing cells unless the cells have been damaged. You are wondering how these cells are damaged? The most common food additive that destroys these critical cells in the hypothalamus is Monosodium Glutamate or MSG. To begin your new eating regime, I recommend you eliminate products that contain these ingredients that may contain MSG; plant protein extract, soy protein, yeast food, whey protein, soy sauce, yeast extract, natural flavors, gelatain, barley malt, broth, bouillon, calcium caseinate, carrageen, autolyzed yeast, hydrolyzed oat flour, hydrolyzed vegetable protein and these are just for starters since there are over forty food ingredients that can contain MSG. It is simpler to look for products that state they are MSG free.

Q:

What does Fair Trade Certified mean that is listed on more and more product labels?

A:

Fair Trade Certified, which began in the mid 1990's, was developed to help consumers support products that are produced on farms that have been certified to provide fair wages, safe working conditions (where forced child labor is prohibited), equal opportunity for advancement, and that healthy working and living conditions are provided for all employees. Fair trade also means environmentally sustainable production and harvest practices and respect for cultural heritage. Current fair trade certified labels can be found on coffee, tea, herbs, cocoa, chocolate, fresh fruit, rice, sugar, flowers, honey and vanilla!

Q:

I love bananas but if I eat too many I seem to have stomach issues, either diarrhea or constipation. Can you please enlighten me on bananas!

A:

Bananas can actually cure diarrhea, cause diarrhea, cause constipation or cure constipation! If you eat green bananas, they can actually help ease constipation since the fiber is highly soluble which can help push the bowel movement through the intestines. On the other hand, too many green bananas, hasten the movement through the bowels more rapidly than is comfortable. Consuming an unripe banana can cause constipation because unripe are high in starch and take a long time to digest. However, ripe bananas contain an enzyme which prevents the fermenting of the banana benefiting anyone that suffers from constipation. Have you ever wondered what the banana peel is good for other than slipping on it? If you suffer from psoriasis, take the inside of the banana peel and rub it over the affected area-you should notice a difference in a few days. The inside of the banana peel also helps on acne. Did you know...Bananas are the world's most popular fruit after tomatoes! The word banana is actually taken from the Arab word "banan" which means finger! Bananas with dark spots on them usually have an higher sugar content than a green banana. Approximately forty four million tons of bananas are produced annually!

Q:

I am a label reader so I stay totally confused when grocery shopping. I recently purchased a product that stated lightly breaded thinking maybe this was healthier but no where on the packaging could I find how "lightly" breaded it was so I guess this is just a marketing statement. Do you know what this means!

A:

There are so many claims on our food items it is confusing to everyone. Here are a few claims: Lightly Sweetened, Good source of....., Reduced Sodium (still contains one hundred and forty milligrams per serving), Natural (USDA has set no definition except on meat & poultry), Reduced Fat, Trans fat free (although it can still contain .49 grams of fat per serving) and the one I dislike the most, Sugar Free (although it usually contains anywhere from three to four genetically modified corn sweeteners). The Lightly Breaded is usually just a distraction, since the product has been rolled in WHITE flour, dipped in some liquid (milk/water), and tossed in a vat of cheap oil with cooking instructions on the package to toss it in the microwave to radiate it. So yes, many claims are just marketing ploys to get the product off the shelf and into your pantry! Keep reading the labels-your health depends on it!

Q:

I have gone back to using butter rather than margarine, for no other reason other than I think it is healthier. Is this something that you would recommend and if so, why?

A:

When you look at the laundry list of ingredients that are listed on the "plastic" margarine tubs, you usually find several ingredients that you are unfamiliar with or cannot even pronounce. Margarine must contain no less than eighty percent fat (those nasty trans fatty acids) along with water, milk solids, salt, preservatives, emulsifiers, artificial colors and flavorings. Margarine is usually made from soy and cottonseed oils, processed under high head, high pressure and uses chemical solvents designed to extract the oil. Butter, on the other hand, is natural, rich in vitamins and minerals, generally wrapped in "paper", in a box and lists it ingredients as just pasteurized cream and salt if you choose that option. Whipped butter is usually found in paper containers as well and the only difference is that it contains about twenty five per cent air. Butter is graded by the FDA (Food and Drug Administration) by taste, color, aroma, texture and body. A score of one hundred is the best, grade AA must score at least a ninety three, grade A at least a ninety two and grade B with a score of a minimum of ninety points. Salt is added to increase shelf life. Based on the processing, packaging and quality, my recommendation will always be butter. Here are a few other tidbits about butter you may find interesting; always use unsalted butter in recipes since the content of salt can range from 1.5% to 3% and can play havoc on your recipe, store butter in a closed container to eliminate the absorption of odors, and if butter is fresh, it will store up to nine months in your freezer. It takes twenty one pounds of whole milk to make one pound of butter! In 2009, more than 1.5 BILLION pounds of butter was produced. I have had butter made from donkey, goat, buffalo, camel and yak (yuk) and I still prefer butter from cows!

Q:

I have candida and was told by my doctor changing my diet could help tremendously and suggested that I contact you for recommendations. I hope you can give me guidance and a simple plan to follow.

A:

Candidiasis or Candida Albicans, is one of several types of fungi that live or grow inside most human bodies according to Dr. James F. Balch. While the body is designed to keep bacteria/ fungi under control, factors can cause the friendly bacteria to die, leaving candida to grow uncontrollably in all or parts of the body. Some symptoms of overgrowth of candida are persistent fatigue, headaches, cough, congestion, poor memory, poor concentration, chronic skin rashes, pain, genital or toenail fungus, allergies, canker sores and kidney/bladder infections. The fungus that causes candidiasis thrives on sugar, yeast, caffeine, glutinous foods (foods that contain gluten), aged cheese and fruit (fresh and dried) so these food should be eliminated from the diet. Foods that are the most beneficial in detoxifying the system are garlic, chlorella, spirulina, and wheatgrass. Alkaline water is beneficial in helping flush yeast toxins out of the system as well. Consuming at least one to two teaspoons of ground Salba or flaxseed daily is important since these have antifungal properties. Meals should be based around vegetables, gluten free grains and lean protein such as fish, organic poultry, lentils and beans. A good whole food, pure, multi vitamin provides the many nutrients used to support detoxification and should also be taken daily. If you choose a yogurt, make sure your selection is unsweetened and contains live yogurt cultures. And last, but perhaps the most important, chronic stress can alter flora balance and suppress the immune system so try to eliminate as much stress as possible.

Q:

What is the difference between a probiotic and a prebiotic?

A:

Probiotics work in the system to balance the potentially dangerous effects of harmful bacteria and aid in digestion. The living organisms that we are most familiar with that a probiotic contains are lactobacillus, acidophilus and bifidobacterium. Probiotics strengthen the gastrointestinal tract lining and can boost the immune system. Probiotics and prebiotics work together as synbiotics. Probiotics do not stimulate metabolic activity whereas prebiotics do. However prebiotics do not contain living organisms like the probiotics, but support the growth and function of those bacteria. Prebiotics are non-absorbable carbohydrates known as fructo and oligo saccharides found in grains, fruits and legumes. One thought to remember is there is little point to send in replacements troops of probiotics if one continues to eat toxic, genetically modified, microwaved foods that destroyed the originals in the beginning!

Q:

Can you please explain what a food label means when is says "Fortified"? I was recently faced with this decision while holding a "plain" juice and one that said "fortified". No where did the product indicate that the fortified was a healthier choice and that made me wonder exactly what it meant. Thank you for your thoughts on this one!

A:

Fortified food means that vitamins and minerals have been added to the food. Sounds good-correct? However, the reason that the vitamins and minerals were added is because all of the nutrients that were originally in the product were lost during the initial processing and refining of the item. To make up for the loss of nutrients, vitamins and minerals are added to "enhance" the nutritional value of the food. Quite often these added nutrients are synthetic and will not be absorbed by the system anyway. As an example, iron might be added to a food, but in some forms it is insoluble and the body will just flush it out without utilizing any of the added iron. I applaud your keen observation of the package wording since it can be very confusing. If you notice, organic food does not state that a product is fortified.

Q:

Why are some eggs brown, some white and some actually look like they have a green hue? Does the color affect the nutrients? Is it true that all organic eggs are brown?

A:

The color of the egg shell usually depends on the breed of chicken; chickens with white earlobes like the White Leghorn breed, will lay white eggs. The Rhode Island Red breed of chicken has red earlobes and will lay brown eggs. Eggs that are green or blue in color are from the Chilean breed of chicken called the Aracuana. While there is some debate whether the original color of eggs was brown or white, we do know that years of cross breeding has resulted in the different colors. The yolk color is directly related to the diet of the chicken with a darker yolk usually indicating a healthier diet although the nutrient level is equal in all eggs. It does appear that most eggs referred to as free range, cage free, or organic are brown eggs. An interesting note is that regardless of the color of the egg, the inside of the shell is always white?

Q:

I do not use artificial sweeteners, but am confused about xylitol, which is considered a natural sweetener. Can you please tell me what I need to look for when purchasing xylitol?

A:

It is very important to know what to look for when purchasing xylitol (zi-lo-tal). There are two sources of xylitol, corn or birch. Because most corn products are genetically modified, it is important to search for a xylitol product that is made from organic birch trees and is made in the United States, since most corn based xylitol is manufactured in China. It is also important to know if the xylitol is pharmaceutical grade. Xylitol from a birch source, pharmaceutical grade and made in the United States is more expensive that the inferior imported variety. However, when your health is at stake, one thing to remember is to never give up quality for cost. An easy way to determine if the xylitol you are considering is manufactured in China is to look at the bar code on the product. If the first three numbers in the bar code begin with 690-695, China is the country of origin and I would recommend NOT purchasing that product! For a full list of product codes, please visit my web site, www.docphyl.com.

Q:

I have fingernails that split continuously and wonder if nutritional deficiencies could be the cause. I am trying to change my diet and lifestyle so I welcome any recommendations.

A:

Nails reveal a lot about our internal health. Here is a list of nutritional deficiencies that can result in nail problems. A deficiency of vitamin A and calcium causes dryness and brittleness, while a deficiency of the B vitamins, especially biotin, causes fragility with horizontal and vertical ridges. Spoon nails are the result of an iron deficiency while those white spots on your nails are the result of a zinc deficiency. If your nails have white bands on them, that indicates a possible protein deficiency. Insufficient intake of vitamin B12 can leave your nails very curved and rounded at the nail ends and very dark. A lack of friendly bacteria in the gut is indicated in nails that have a fungus under and around the nails or splitting nails that could indicate an insufficient amount of hydrochloric acid in the stomach. For splitting nails or hangnails, take two tablespoons of brewer's yeast or wheat germ oil daily, and as I always recommend, take a whole food supplement daily with plenty of good, clean alkaline water.

Q:

My daughter has been diagnosed with fructose intolerance. It took us some time to figure out why she was suffering from bloating, abdominal cramps, gas and diarrhea. I took her off of milk and that helped tremendously but the problem still persisted. Now that we have more direction, I would appreciate any information about this disorder and possibly a list of foods that she should avoid since I am unfamiliar with this.

A:

There are actually two types of fructose intolerance that exist. One is Hereditary Fructose Intolerance (HFI) or fructose poisoning, which is a rare genetic disorder and is very serious. Hereditary fructose intolerance is a condition where individuals lack a liver enzyme, adolase b, that allows the body to break down fructose during digestion and can become serious enough to affect the liver and kidneys. The second form of fructose intolerance is actually known as fructose malabsorption and is a condition where individuals simply have difficulty digesting fructose as is the case with your daughter. Fructose is the sugar naturally found in fruits and should be avoided. It is also important to avoid all man made fructose such as high fructose corn syrup and sorbitol. The following should also be avoided: table sugar (sucrose), confectioner's sugar or powdered sugar, fruit juices (fresh squeezed, tinned or bottled), honey, sodas, flavored water, sports drinks, coconut milk, stevia, molasses, sweetened milk or sweetened milk beverages and dried fruit. For a full list, please visit my web site, www.docphyl.com.

Q:

I recently read an article about what vegetables and fruits contain more pesticides than others? I found the article interesting and thought you might share this information with your readers.

A:

Thank you for sharing your concerns about pesticide toxicity in our produce. Some produce is more susceptible to pests and therefore require more pesticides to eliminate damage to the produce. It is important to remember than not only can pesticides contaminate the skin of the vegetable or fruit, it can also be absorbed into the meat of the produce. According to the Environmental Working Group, the list of produce that contains the *least* amount of pesticides includes: onions, avocado, sweet corn, pineapple, mango, asparagus, sweet peas, cabbage, kiwi, eggplant, papaya, watermelon, broccoli, tomato, and sweet potato. The list of produce that contains the *highest* amount of pesticides includes: peaches, apples, celery, nectarines, sweet bell peppers, strawberries, cherries, lettuce, grapes, pears, spinach and potatoes.

Q:

Can you please tell me why some beans cause me to have so much gas and others do not! It is embarrassing.

A:

The problem with flatulence, or what we casually call gas, is produced by the fermentation of the complex sugar oligosaccharide found in beans and some other vegetables, such as cabbage and broccoli. The small intestine does not have the proper enzyme to break this sugar down but as it passes into the large intestine, bacteria breaks it down and unfortunately ferments the sugar producing hydrogen, methane and carbon dioxide gases. The following list was released by the USDA's Western Laboratory in

Berkley, California. The list is in order of those beans that produce the most gas, based on the beans sugar content, to the beans that contain the lowest amount of sugar and therefore produce the least amount of gas. Number one is soybeans that are rated ten (which may require a gas mask) pea beans rated nine, black beans rated 8.5, pinto beans also rated at 8.5 (which may still clear out the house), california small white beans rated 8, Great Northern beans rated a seven, lima beans rated 6.5, garbanzos beans (chick peas) rated six and black eyed-peas rated five. The flatulence problem was studied among pilots since gas expands at higher altitudes causing gut discomfort. At thirty five thousand feet, gas will expand to 5.4 times more than at sea level. In the 1960's, astronauts were selected based on the individuals that produced the least amount of gas. The beans that caused the biggest problems were found to be navy and lima beans with pinto beans trailing in at third place.

Q:

What does the word "parve" mean that is listed on food packages. Sometimes I see it with different letters in front on the word. Please explain!

A:

"Parve" or "pareve" is used to identify Kosher food and means neutral. By Jewish customs, that means that a product is neither meat nor diary, has not been cooked or mixed with any meat or diary and that it does not contain any meat derivatives. This also means that the food product is suitable for vegetarians and is considered one hundred percent dairy free and therefore safe for someone that is following a strict casein free diet. The circle around the letter represents the letter "O" for Orthodox. If the circle contains the letter K before the word parve, that means that the product is Kosher and if there is a U circled in front of parve, that stands for Union.

Q:

Are there foods that can help lower cholesterol and triglycerides?

A:

If you are concerned about your cholesterol and triglycerides, have changed your dietary lifestyle to choosing healthier foods and incorporating more exercise, here are a few suggestions for you to consider with your doctor's permission. Artichoke extract, barley, psyllium, green tea extract (decaf, of course) and oat bran, may be helpful in reducing cholesterol. Fish oil, ground flaxseed, Salba seed and garlic extract can be beneficial in reducing triglycerides. One very popular choice for lowering cholesterol and LDL cholesterol, according to the Mayo Clinic web site, is red yeast rice. Red yeast rice is the product of yeast grown on rice and is served as a dietary supplements in some Asian countries. Red yeast rice contains several compounds collectively know as monacolins known to inhibit cholesterol synthesis. For more information regarding red yeast rice, visit the web site of mayoclinic.com and webmd.com.

Q:

I notice from time to time that when I break an egg, there is a red bloody looking spot in the egg that I find disgusting. I have learned to crack the egg in a separate bowl to prevent ruining my ingredients that I am preparing. What causes this and is it unsafe to eat?

A:

Occasionally red spots can be found in eggs. As the yolk membrane travels down the reproductive track, before it is surrounded by the albumen, it is possible for a small drop of blood to attach itself to the yolk. The blood may be the result of a small arterial rupture or from some other source of bleeding. It does not indicate that fertilization has taken place and if the egg is properly cooked it is not harmful. If you feel uncomfortable with the blood spot, you can easily remove it with a knife tip of a piece of the egg shell. Egg manufacturing use a process called candling, when the eggs are rolled over high intensity lights which can detect the red spots and those eggs are normally removed. Less than one percent of eggs with the blood spot, may slip through the candling process, so called because in the beginning of egg inspections, the egg was simply held up to a candle to detect abnormalities.

Q:

I have noticed that my non-stick skillet coating is peeling and flaking off so I am going to get rid of it. I have done a little bit of research on different coatings and now I wonder if I even want to replace it with another one or use something different. What is the coating made of and can it be dangerous? Can you please shed some light on this subject for me?

A:

While the non-stick pans seem to be a wonderful kitchen tool, research indicates that it may not be so good after all. In 2006, the Environmental Protection Agency (EPA), asked eight American companies to work toward the elimination of perfluorooctanoic acid (PFOA) a chemical used to bond non-stick coatings to the pan, by 2015. The EPA labeled PFOA's as a likely carcinogen since PFOA's have been shown to cause cancer, low birth weights and suppressed immune systems in laboratory animals exposed to high levels of PFOA'S. Once food is cooked above certain temperatures, hotter than the smoke point of oils, non-stick coating will break down and release toxins. I would recommend that you toss the cookware if it is peeling or chipping and grab you a cast iron skillet. The odds are those black specs in your scrambled eggs are not pepper!

Q:

I recently had an attack of severe pain in my big toe that was diagnosed as gout. A friend suggested that I drink some black cherry juice. I was amazed at how it helped. Can you please explain what is in black cherry juice that helped me so much!

A:

Gout, a very painful form of arthritis, is caused by high levels of uric acid in the system that result in inflammation, swelling and redness at the affected area. Black cherry juice contains anthocyanin, a chemical that naturally helps relieve inflammation. Anthocyanins are plant based compounds that contain high levels of antioxidants and are the pigments responsible for the red, purple and blue colors in fruits and vegetables. The top anthocyanin containing foods are Black Currant, Blackberry, Blueberry, Chokeberry, Cranberry, Black Cherry and the grand poo-pah of all -can you guess it-EGGPLANT!!! There are seven hundred milligrams of anthocyanins in a 100 gram serving of Eggplant!

Q:

Can you please tell me the fastest way to ripen an avocado? I am not the best a picking a ripe avocado and find myself ready to use it and it is not ready! Any suggestions?

A:

The fastest way to ripen an avocado is to place it in a wool sock and set it in the back of a dark closet for two days! If you are not in to big of a hurry, avocados will also ripen if placed in a brown paper bag and set in a warm location. Depending on the state of ripeness, sometimes adding a banana to the sock or bag will also speed up the process! It is best to NOT store an avocado in the refrigerator unless it is fully ripe. (P.S. Don't forget you put the avocado in the sock in your closet or you will wonder why it smells like guacamole every time you open the door!)

Q:

What is cream of tartar? It is true that you can use it for cooking and household cleaning?

A:

Tartar is derived from grapes during and after the fermentation process. After wine has been fermented, two mauve colored crystalline sediments remain in the wine casks. The sediment that collects on the sides of the wine cask is called "argols" and the sediment that settles on the bottom of the cask is called "lees". These two substances are actually crude tartar. The crude tartar is then de-crystallized by cooking in boiling water which allows the remains to crystallize again. The remaining substance is then bleached pure white and crystallized again. As this process concludes, a very thin like layer of white crystals is formed on the surface. The name "cream of tartar" is derived from this thin top layer that actually resembles the look of cream. It is used to produce baking powder when mixed with baking soda. Cream of tartar is the common name for potassium hydrogen tartrate which is an acidic salt and can be used to clean copper and brass cookware. Cream of tartar combined with hydrogen peroxide is excellent for cleaning tough rust stains!

Q:

What is the animal source of the milk used in making Roquefort cheese and why does it smell so strong?

A:

Roquefort cheese is a blue cheese made from raw, unpasteurized, not homogenized ewe's (sheep) milk which is curdled with calf rennet. The pungent smell to cheese is the bacteria. Spores of fungus Penicillium roqueforti are added to vats of the heated ewe's milk which allows the milk to ferment into solids called curds. When the curds are ready, they are cubed and placed in cheese molds where they are drained of the liquid (whey) and salted. These cheese molds are then pierced throughout approximately fifty times to allow air to enter and mold fungus to grow before being transferred to Cambalou caves for natural ripening. The cheese loaves are left exposed for two to three weeks. Once enough penicillium roqueforti has grown within the cheese loaves, they are wrapped and left for the duration, as long as ten months, before exiting the cave as Roquefort cheese and its distinct flavor and strong smell!

Q:

I am not a breakfast eater-is that a good thing or not?

A:

Breakfast is a compound word that means break and fast. Hence breakfast is important to **break** the **fast** the body has endured during your sleeping hours. After a night of rebuilding, the body needs to be replenished and refueled with water (rather than caffeine) and food, preferably protein and fiber rather than sugary, high calorie, over processed foods. If you skip breakfast, your body goes as long as fifteen to twenty hours before a mid-day meal which creates a period of semistarvation resulting in physical, intellectual and behavioral problems according to webmd. Research indicates that skipping meals, especially breakfast, can actually make losing weight more difficult. Those individuals that skip breakfast have a tendency to eat more at the next meal and snack more throughout the day. For those that eat breakfast every day, they generally choose healthier foods throughout the day. "Eat breakfast like a King, lunch like a Prince and dinner like a Pauper" as quoted by Adelle Davis.

Q:

Why do apples float? How many varieties of apples are there and why should I eat an apple a day?

A:

Fresh apples float because twenty five percent of their volume is air! There are a total of approximately seven thousand five hundred varieties of apples around the world, twenty five hundred of those varieties are grown here in the United States! Eating an apple a day is a wonderful benefit to the body because of the fiber (if you eat the skin) and because apples contain pectin-a natural toxin eliminator. Here are a few other facts about apples that you might find interesting; Apples do not contain fat, sodium or cholesterol. Apples are covered with a natural layer of wax we call the skin. The skin actually protects all the liquid the apple naturally contains. In fact, because of all of that liquid, it takes only thirty six apples to make a gallon of apple cider. China is the leading producer of apples with over 1.2 billion bushels grown yearly.

Q:

Tell me about pumpkins? Are they a fruit or a vegetable?

A:

With the wonderful days of autumn upon us, pumpkin season is around the corner. Pumpkins are in the vine crop family called cucurbits, therefore they are considered a fruit rather than a vegetable (uh oh-did some of you get that one wrong?) The name "pumpkin" originated from the Greek word "pepon" which means "large melon". The French changed the word to "pompon". The English changed "pompon" to "Pumpion" then to "Ponpions" and the American colonist changed the word to pumpkin. Whew! Pumpkins contain approximately ninety percent water. Eighty percent of the supply of pumpkins in the United States is in October with almost ninety five percent of the processed pumpkins grown in Illinois. The health benefits of pumpkins are enormous. That bright orange color is an indicator that the fruit is loaded with beta carotene, a very beneficial carotenoid converted to Vitamin A in the body. Just one cup of pumpkin contains approximately two thousand six hundred and fifty IU's (international units) of Vitamin A. Pumpkins are low in fat and sodium, and high in fiber and protein and are an excellent source of B vitamins and iron! And don't forget those pumpkin seeds! They are also a wonderful source of vitamins and minerals. If you suffer from "Apocolocynposis", you may not have enjoyed this column! That is the fear of turning into a pumpkin!

Q:

Do food colorings contain toxic metals? I have a child with ADHD and I am trying to eliminate as many toxics from our diet as possible and food coloring seems to be in everything.

A:

Lead, mercury and arsenic are all ingredients used in most artificial food colorings. FD&C Red #3 contains lead and arsenic while FD&C Yellow #5 contains all three, lead, mercury and arsenic. The Academy of Child and Adolescent Psychiatry estimates that one out of every six children in the United States has blood levels in the toxic range. The Journal of Environmental Health Perspectives recently published an article that stated children with blood lead levels more than two micrograms per deciliter were four times more likely to be diagnosed with ADHD (Attention Deficit Hyperactivity Disorder). While sports drinks, cereals, lotions, and shampoos may contain food coloring, pesticides on fruits and vegetables may also contain arsenic, lead, copper, mercury and other toxic metals. Hydrogenated oils may contain nickel and cadmium which are used as catalysts. Table salt has aluminum added as an anti caking agent, which is why so many now prefer sea salt. It is important to be label savvy when purchasing products and search out the food coloring which is buried somewhere in the laundry list of ingredients. Here is a bit of FYI (for your information): Food coloring Red #3 has had a proposed ban on it from the FDA in the past after the dye was linked to thyroid tumors in experimental testing. The FDA had the dye removed from external drugs and cosmetics. For a complete list of all metals found in ingredients, topical and consumable, go the FDA (Food and Drug Administration) website.

Q:

I see Xanthan Gum listed as an ingredient quite often but I recently came across a recipe that called for Xanthan gum. What is it exactly?

A:

Xanthan gum is a polysaccharide used as a food additive and rheology modifier or in simpler terms, a thickening agent and emulsifier. Xanthan gum is an excellent source of dietary fiber and can be used by individuals that suffer from celiac disease which is a sensitivity to wheat gluten. That is why Xanthan gum is listed in so many gluten free products and recommended in gluten free recipes. Xanthan gum is free of sugar, starch, soy, yeast, wheat, corn, milk and salt.

Q:

My family has recently quit drinking regular cow's milk and my children's allergies and stomach issues have improved tremendously. I am searching for a good substitute that is healthy, but am confused when I start looking and comparing. Can you please give me some nutritional values on milk substitutes?

A:

There are many that are "udderly" confused about milk and non diary substitutes so hopefully this will help! The casein in cow's milk is designed to be digested by a calf, not humans, which is why we develop so many digestive problems and allergies when drinking cow's milk. Soy milk contains phytoestrogens and quite often uses hexan (a toxin) in its processing which is why it can be eliminated rather quickly as a non diary substitute. That leaves Almond, Rice, Oat, Hemp and Coconut as safe non-diary "milk" substitutes. For many, it is a taste choice as each has their unique flavor! If you are looking for the lowest calorie content, Almond would be the choice. Per cup, Almond "milk" contains only sixty calories compared to Rice "milk" that contains one hundred and twenty calories, Oat and Hemp "milk" contain one hundred and thirty, and Coconut "milk" contains five hundred and fifty two calories! Almond also contains the lowest sugar content per serving, seven grams. While coconut does have the highest calorie content, it also contains the highest iron content, twenty two percent, and the lowest sodium content of all non diary substitutes at thirty six percent. Almond and Oat "milk" contain the lowest fat percentage of any of the non diary products around two percent. All of these percentages are approximate depending on the brand and if they are unsweetened, which will drop the total calorie count. Non diary substitute drinks are from natural, raw nuts and seeds and are sold in tetra pak (paper) containers rather than plastic. While most of the non diary "milk" products are lactose free, cholesterol free, and gluten free I recommend that you DO NOT use non diary substitutes in an infant formula.

Q:

Is there a nutritional value difference between steel cut oats and regular rolled oats?

A:

Serving for serving, they are equal in calories, carbohydrates, fiber, sugar and protein. The only difference is the fat content which is .05 grams more for rolled oats that steel cut. Both have a low glycemic index (the rate of increase in blood sugar levels after a food is eaten). Rolled oats are rolled flat while steel cut are whole oats cut into small chunks. Steel cuts oats are chewier, have a nutty flavor and take the edge on processing since they are not steamed like rolled oats are. Steel cut oats take twice as long to cook than rolled oats.

Q:

Can you please give me some facts about the evaporated milk versus condensed milk?

A:

Evaporated milk is made from fresh non-pasteurized whole milk that is then processed, in its can, at temperatures over two hundred degrees to sterilize it. This results in somewhat of a burnt taste that can be eliminated by mixing it into a recipe. Condensed milk, on the other hand, does not require high heat sterilization since it contains over forty percent sugar, which acts as a preservative, thus reducing bacterial growth. Did you know that the stability of evaporated milk can be improved by stirring in one tablespoon of lemon juice to one cup of milk? Also, if you do not use the entire can of evaporated milk, transfer the remainder into a well sealed glass jar and refrigerate. Did you know that condensed milk contains a whopping nine hundred and eighty calories per eight ounces, and that it can be stored at room temperature for up to six months? Condensed milk cannot be substituted for evaporated milk in recipes.

Q:

Are there seeds other than apple seeds that contain cyanide? If you consume too many seeds that contain cyanide, what are the symptoms?

A:

Apricot, peach, plum, cherry and pear seeds also contain cyanogenic acids ! While apple seeds do contain cyanide, the poison is encased in a seed that cannot be broken down by the body's digestive system and is therefore harmlessly excreted! (I do recommend that you DO NOT place a whole apple in the blender if you juice-remove the core first). If you accidently swallow a few seeds, you will absorb a minimal amount of the toxin. However, if you chew the seeds and accidently swallow some, you are more likely to suffer poisoning. Symptoms of mild poisoning include headaches, confusion, dizziness, vomiting and anxiety. More severe symptoms include elevated blood pressure, elevated heart rate and difficulty breathing. I always recommend that you avoid chewing the seeds of these fruits!

Q:

Can you please tell me if there is a simple way to test my vitamins to see if they are good ones? If so, have you tested yours?

A:

Vitamins and minerals sometimes fail to dissolve in the body, usually due to a poor quality of ingredients and manufacturing practices that are less than desirable. Here is a simple way to test your supplements; heat equal parts of vinegar (any type) and water to approximately one hundred degrees and maintain that temperature (using a glass coffee pot works great). Place your supplement in the solution, occasionally stirring, but being careful not to touch the supplement. If your supplement does not dissolve within forty five minutes, it will more than likely NOT dissolve in your digestive system. The reason it should take so long is the nutrients need to finish dissolving in the small intestine to be properly absorbed. The supplements that I take dissolved in approximately thirty minutes. There is no need to try this on chewable vitamins or time released products for obvious reasons.

Q:

Is coffeeberry decaffeinated?

A:

Coffeeberry is the bright red fruit on the coffee plant that contains the coffee bean. In previous processing of the coffee bean, the red fruit outer casing was discarded because it molded quickly and produced toxins. Because of safe, new technology, the red skin of the coffee plant can be produced safely which is a breakthrough since the red skin contains so many nutrients, including high levels of phenolic acid. Phenolic acids are essential constituents of polyphenols, which are antioxidants! Because the caffeine containing bean grows inside the coffeeberry, there is a trace amount of caffeine in the final product. While the coffeeberry cannot be "claimed" to be one hundred percent caffeine free, (neither can decaffeinated coffees-they are only 99.7% caffeine free), it is generally referred to as a decaffeinated product because it contains less than two percent of caffeine per serving.

Q:

Since you are a food trivia buff, I have a question that is somewhat nutritional, or at least it has to do with food. Whose is Betty Crocker? I see her products but never see a picture like we do Colonel Sanders or Aunt Jemima. Can you explain?

A:

To publicize Gold Medal flour after it became a General Mills product, a picture puzzle ad was run in a national magazine. The company was inundated with over 30,000 people responding to the puzzle and asking questions like "How do you make a one-crust cherry pie?" And "What's a good recipe for apple dumplings?" The advertising staff was bewildered but it rose to the occasion. Recipes from laboratory personnel, home economists, office personnel and their wives were collected and each letter received a personal reply. Each response was simply signed; ***Sincerely***! People then replied with thank you's for the great recipes but had no name to address the thank you to and began asking who was sending the wonderful recipes. Once again the marketing staff rose to the occasion. They came up with a surname, Crocker-the last name of a gentleman that was a long time staff member that had recently retired. Now all they needed was a cozy first name and Betty had the appeal and sounded good with Crocker. Thereafter all letters were signed- Sincerely, Betty Crocker! Today over one hundred women help maintain the Betty Crocker tradition. Five specially trained correspondents answer her personnel mail with well over five thousand letters a month, and a staff to operate nineteen fully equipped kitchens to test over fifty thousand recipes each year. And now you know the rest of the story!

Q:

I have stomach problems and someone recently recommended that I try aloe vera. Can you please explain any benefits of aloe vera?

A:

Aloe vera, is quite often referred to a the lily of the desert. Aloe is a potent healing superfood with a wealth of new research being revealed daily. At this time, there have been over seventy-five healing compounds that have been identified in aloe as well as the fact that aloe has excellent transdermal properties allowing it to penetrate deep skin levels. Aloe gel has been used as far back since Egyptian times as a healer for cuts, burns, insect bites, sores, acne, eczema and burns. Aloe juice has become popular since it boosts the body's cleansing action, balancing rather than causing harsh irritant effects. Aloe juice has anti-inflammatory essential fatty acids that help the stomach and the colon. Aloe juice alkalizes the digestive processes to prevent an over acid system which is a common cause of indigestion and acid reflux and can benefit other stomach and digestive tract irritations like colitis and irritable bowel syndrome. As I always recommend, be sure to tell your physician of any personal protocols that you are taking.

Q:

I read an article that stated that the human body stores between four hundred to eight hundred toxic chemicals. A study conducted by Columbia School of Public Health stated that ninety five percent of cancers can be attributed to diet and environmental toxicity. Is there a list of toxins that we should avoid to lessen our risk of developing cancer? Can you please share your thoughts and a list of toxins in our foods and our environment?

A:

Here is a list of what I will refer to as the top toxins and what they are contained in whether it be a food or environment. This list is by no means all inclusive since there are over seventy seven thousand chemicals produced in North America, over three thousand chemicals added to our food, over nine thousand chemical preservatives, emulsifiers and solvents used in food processing and many more new chemicals introduced each year. Below is a list of the most prevalent toxins that are circulating in our food, water and air supply. ***Polychlorinated Biphenyls*** that are referred to as PCB's which has been banned in the United States but is still present in our environment. ***Pesticides***, according to the Environmental Protection Agency (EPA) sixty percent of herbicides, ninety percent of fungicides and thirty percent of insecticides are known to be carcinogenic. ***Molds***, from contaminated buildings, can cause a wide range of health problems from a small of amount of exposure. ***Phthalates*** are chemicals used to lengthen the life of fragrances and soften plastics. Primary sources are plastic wraps, plastic bottles and plastic food containers. ***Volatile Organic Compounds***, that according to the EPA, are in more indoor air because they are present in numerous household products like varnishes, cosmetics, moth repellents and air fresheners. ***Dioxins***, are chemical compounds that are the result of waste incineration and from burning fuels. ***Asbestos***, although no longer used, is still in old insulation of floors, in ceilings, and in water pipes used between the 1950's and the 1970's. ***Heavy Metals*** like arsenic, mercury, lead, aluminum and cadmium that are in our water supply, vaccines, pesticides and deodorants. ***Chloroform***, a colorless liquid found in our air, drinking water and foods. And ***Chlorine***, one of the most heavily used chemical agents. This highly toxic gas is found in household cleaners, drinking water and in the air near industrial process plants that use chlorine. Remember that most of these toxins you cannot see, smell or feel. It is important to read labels on all products and try to avoid those that contain any of the above toxins, Although I can't list all seventy seven thousand toxins, this list is a great start! Do you know where toxins store themselves in the human body? In our fat cells and in the soft tissue! Now you know why you feel so good after a deep tissue massage-you have released a lot of toxic chemicals.

Q:

I know that nutrients are critical for the human body every day which is why they are called essential. Please tell me exactly what the body does in a twenty four hour period that nutrients in the form of daily supplements can help with?

A:

Because our food lacks in nutrients it is important to take a good whole food supplement to help your body through a twenty four hour period as it regenerates. What happens exactly: on average your heart beats 103, 689 times, your lungs respire 23, 045 times, your blood flows 16,800 miles, your nails grow .00007 inches, your hair grows .01715 inches, you breathe 438 cubic feet of air daily, you speak 4,800 words (women speak more than men-but you knew that already-right?) you take in 3.25 pounds of food and another 2.9 pounds of liquid and you move approximately 25.4 times during your sleep at night! No wonder you feel tired!!

Q:

I have been diagnosed with Ankylosing Spondylitis. Can you please make some diet suggestions?

A:

Ankylosing Spondylitis is a chronic condition, and a form of arthritis resulting in joint pain and inflammation primarily in the spine and pelvis region. It is recommended to eat plenty of vegetables, some fruits, garlic- which helps with inflammation, beet root, coconut water and coconut milk. It is important to follow a low starch diet, based on research by rheumatologist Dr. Alan Ebringer. Dr. Ebringer's belief is that ankylosing spondylitis is caused by a bacteria that resides in the stomach, and that starchy foods promotes the bacteria's growth, therefore removal of starchy foods can eliminate it. It is also recommended to eliminate sugar and caffeine. If you smoke, it is imperative to quit as soon as possible. I would suggest that you eliminate nightshades from the diet. Nightshades include tomatoes, potatoes, peppers and eggplant. Nightshades are reputed by some to cause or worsen arthritis and ankylosing spondylitis. Men are ten times more likely to develop ankylosing spondylitis than women and do so between the ages of 20 to 40. Ever wonder why Ed Sullivan had a different physique-he suffered from Ankylosing Spondylitis!

Q:

I have suffered with migraines for years but it seems like they are becoming more frequent and some are more severe than others. I have read that foods can be a cause but I can never find a list of what is in a food product that may trigger a migraine. All of us migraine suffers thank you for your help.

A:

A host of foods contain chemicals that can cause headaches, including that one-sided, throbbing headache known as a migraine. Here is a list of food additives that should be avoided to reduce the risk of developing migraines : 1) MSG, monosodium glutamate, is a flavor enhancer used in restaurants and in prepared foods such as soups, salad dressings, and lunchmeats that can provoke severe headaches as well as causing flushing and tingling of the head and should be avoided by a headache prone individual. 2) Nitrites, which are preservatives, are commonly found in hot dogs, bacon, salami, and other cured meats. 3) Caffeine, which can act as a vasoconstrictor, and as a result, limit blood flow through the blood vessels in your head and should be avoided in you suffer from migraines. While the experts are divided regarding caffeine, I always recommend avoiding any products that contain caffeine. 4) Aspartame, an artificial sweetener, should be avoided at all extremes. One of the most frequent complaints of food products to the FDA is aspartame. 5) Tyramine, an amino acid, is found in aged cheeses, pickled herring, chicken livers, canned figs, fresh baked goods made with yeast, lima beans, Italian beans, lentils, snow peas, navy beans, pinto beans, peanuts, sunflower seeds, pumpkin seeds and sesame seeds. An astounding thirty percent of migraine sufferers seem to have a sensitivity to tyramine according to Dr. Seymour Diamond, M.D. of the National Headache Foundation. 6) Phenylethylamine, a chemical found in chocolates, can also cause headaches. And 7) Congeners, are chemicals found in hard liquor, and should also be avoided.

Q:

My 27 year old daughter has had surgery twice for kidney stones. She was advised by her physician to eliminate high calcium foods from her diet. My concern is that a low calcium diet will put her at high risk for osteoporosis. Would you comment?

A:

A low calcium diet can increase the risk of developing osteoporosis, an abnormal loss of bone that can lead to fractures in later years. Your daughter's chances of avoiding osteoporosis will improve if she exercises regularly, doesn't smoke, avoids heavy intake of alcohol and eliminates caffeine. There is evidence that low calcium diets can increase the frequency of kidney stones whereas high calcium diets can do the opposite. This seeming paradox may have to do with the effect of dietary calcium in preventing the absorption of oxalates from the intestine.

Q:

Can you please explain exactly what SALBA is and what the health benefits are! Is SALBA related to the chia seed?

A:

Salba is a 100% natural antique South American grain that was first used by the Aztec civilization and its roots dates back as early as 3500 B.C.. Salba is a variety of the Salvia hispanica L. botanical family of mint called chia! Although SALBA comes from chia, it is not the exact same substance, as SALBA has more nutritional value than chia. Salba is all natural, contains no trans fats, is completely gluten free, contains very few carbohydrates and is certified non-GMO (NOT genetically modified organism). Since SALBA is gluten free, it makes an excellent substitute for flour (1 part SALBA replaces three parts flour). Gram for gram, SALBA contains fifteen times more magnesium than broccoli, eight times more omega-3 than salmon, six times more calcium than milk, three times more iron than spinach and three times more antioxidant strength than blueberries! Best of all, SALBA has the perfect balance of omega-3 and omega-6 fatty acids found in nature. SALBA holds a United States medical patent and is the only whole food in existence that is medically patented.

Q:

Can I eat green bananas?

A:

Green bananas are safe to eat even though they can be bitter when eaten raw! Some studies even suggest that green bananas are healthier than their yellow counterpart! Green bananas contain a resistant starch called short fatty chain (SCFAs) which is helpful for people controlling their blood sugar. Green bananas also offer diabetics a high energy, low calorie source of carbohydrates which meets their dietary restrictions. According to the National Institutes of Health, SCFAs enhances the body's capacity to absorb nutrients. The incidence of IBS (Irritable Bowel Disease) and cancers is lower in places where people consume more green bananas than yellow!

My recommendation is to slice the green bananas and sauté them in butter! UMMM, MMMM, Good and healthy!

Q:

Can you please explain the difference between "sustainably caught" and "wild caught" and "farm raised" fish? I am totally confused about which is the best purchase!

A:

According to Greenpeace, a fish is **Sustainable** if it comes from a fishery with practices than can be maintained indefinitely without reducing the species' ability to maintain its population without adversely impacting other species within the ecosystem by removing their food source, accidently killing them or damaging their physical environment. **Wild caught** fish are hatchery spawned fish-fish that have been farm raised then released into the ocean to be caught. **Farm raised fish**, the product of aquaculture, are fish raised in large, underwater cages and in many cases injected with growth hormones. The practice of farm raised fish started as a reaction to our fishing practices that caused many fish species such as halibut, cod, orange roughy and sea bass to become depleted. Of late, criticism is being raised of farm raised fishing practices because fish are too crowded in the cages, fed too many antibiotics and growth hormones and dyes are being added to the water leaving it toxic, and the fish are being exposed to and absorbing these chemicals. Fish naturally spawned, grown in the wild and caught in the wild are still the best catch!

Q:

I do not drink milk but do enjoy a bowl of granola occasionally and wonder what is the best non-dairy "milk" substitute; soy milk, almond milk, coconut milk or rice milk?

A:

The best flavour will depend on your palate and the manufacturer. If you prefer a slightly nutty taste, a bit creamy with little or no fat, almond milk is excellent. It is made by pressing the nuts and adding water. Almonds are one of the healthiest nuts you can eat because of their nutrient content and therefore is the most nutritious milk alternative on the market. Soy milk, made by pressing the soybean and adding water, has a good fat content, a decent amount of vitamin B 12, no cholesterol and less fat than regular cow's milk. However, soy has certain properties that can interfere with the body's ability to assimilate nutrients. Coconut milk is actually made by pressing the white meat in the coconut husk while rice milk is made from pre-soaked or dried brown rice and filtered water. Rice milk contains less protein than soy and almond milk.

Q:

Can you please tell me if there are certain fruits and vegetables that absorb or contain more pesticide residue that other fruits and vegetables. My child is over sensitive to chemicals even though we wash what we eat thoroughly. Also, is rinsing with water enough?

A:

There is a list of fruits and vegetables, referred to as the dirty dozen, that have been analyzed for pesticide residue levels from the U.S. Department of Agriculture (USDA). This list is the most common foods with the *highest* levels of pesticide residues. FRUITS: Apples, cherries, grapes (imported), nectarines, pears, peaches, raspberries, strawberries. VEGETABLES: Celery, potatoes, spinach, and bell peppers. Just as an FYI (for your information) here is a list of fruits and vegetables that contain the *least* amount of pesticide residue. FRUITS: Kiwi, mango, bananas, papaya and pineapple. VEGETABLES: Asparagus, avocado, onions, broccoli, cauliflower, peas (sweet), corn (sweet). Washing your fruits and vegetables thoroughly in water is usually ample. Quite often, if you rinse your vegetable in a washing solution, you may not always rinse all of the solution off and that can in turn cause stomach upset.

Q:

I recently purchased a product that said "no trans fats". When I got home, I read the label more thoroughly and saw that it listed partially hydrogenated fat. How can it say no trans fats with a hydrogenated product in the list of ingredients?

A:

Food labels can be very misleading. What the label is missing is the wording "PER SERVING". When the law became effective in 2006 that a food product label indicate the trans fat it contained, manufactures simply reduced the serving size. So even though the product still contains the heart damaging trans fats, the serving size is so small, the claim may be made. Any product that contains .05 grams or less of trans fats per serving, is by law, allowed to say "No trans fat (per serving)" Quite often the "per serving" has been omitted. Prior to the law becoming effective I purchased ten products that I knew contained trans fats. After the law was effective, January, 2006, I purchased the exact same products only to find that none of them indicated trans fats on the label. When I looked at the serving size on the products, some servings were dropped as much from a 1 cup serving to a 1 tablespoon serving. The most important wording to look for is hydrogenated or partially hydrogenated on the label and to avoid any product that contains those words.

Q:

I eat a lot of legumes and am always surprised at how many people do not know what legumes are. Any chance you can explain what these are would be appreciated not only by my friends but all of those that do not know what they are!

A:

Legumes are peas, lentils, carob, peanuts and beans including soybean products like soy milk, tofu and tempeh. Legumes grow in pods on vines while peanuts grow underground. Legumes are high in protein, containing between twenty five to thirty eight percent which is more than eggs and many meats, contains no cholesterol or saturated fats and are very high in dietary fiber.

Q:

Can you please explain the difference between flours? I see pastry flour, bread flour, all purpose flour, spelt flour and the like?

A:

All purpose flour is the baker's workhouse in the kitchen. Most contain about eleven to twelve percent protein. What is interesting is that Midwestern and Northern brands usually contain higher protein amounts per serving while in the Southern and Northwestern brands contain lower amounts of protein. If you recipe flops-check the protein amount because if it contains over 13.2 grams per cup you may be in for a disaster and can't figure out why! Pastry flour is a low protein flour containing between 8-9% protein and is usually unbleached. Bleached flour is when mills use chlorine gas to speed up the aging process and peroxide to whiten the flour. Unbleached does not go through this process. Cake flour is a soft, low-protein flour usually containing 7-9% protein which is perfect for a light cake. Bread flour contains 12-13% protein which gives your bread a strong skeletal structure to hold its shape during rising, baking and cutting. Self-rising flour contains baking powder and salt which is excellent for pancakes and biscuits. Spelt flour, is an ancient European grain, that has become popular in the United States with individuals that have sensitivities to traditional wheat. Spelt flour contains protein levels as high as 17% which makes it a great replacement for whole wheat!

Q:

My son has been diagnosed with Autism and I am struggling trying to find nutritional information. I was told that nutrition was important but am getting stressed trying to find nutrition answers about what I can do to help him. Are there certain foods he should avoid that can help with his digestion? I understand nutrition cannot cure Autism but any suggestions you could give me would be greatly appreciated.

A:

Autism is a complex biological developmental disorder. No single cause has been determined at this time although genetic and environmental factors are implicated. You are correct in that nutrition cannot cure Autism, however, there are several nutritional therapies that can benefit a child with Autism. Many parents of Autistic children, report that their children received repeated or prolong treatment of antibiotics for respiratory infections, in their younger years, prior to the Autistic diagnosis by their physician. Because broad-spectrum antibiotics kill good as well as bad bacteria in the gut, restoring a healthy gut is very important. You can start by supplementing with digestive enzymes and giving probiotics to restore balance of gut bacteria. Both of these measures may begin the healing process of the digestive track and promote normal absorption. The strongest link of problem foods to Autism is wheat and diary and the specific proteins they contain, namely gluten and casein, because they are difficult to digest. Milk restriction or near elimination is an ABSOLUTE imperative to the treatment of Autism. COMPLETE elimination of the following foods can also benefit the diet of an Autistic child since quite often they suffer from allergies; sugar, juice, canned sodas, strawberries, French fries, artificial sweeteners, and monosodium glutamate. Avoid anything made with lead or mercury and be diligent in reading food labels, and eliminate foods with a laundry list of ingredients. Remember, if you read an ingredient that you cannot pronounce, place it back on the shelf!

Q:

I am from the new generation but I hear the older generation say ; " An apple a day keeps the doctor away"! Can you please tell why it is so healthy for someone to eat an apple daily? Do you have a favorite?

A:

The old proverb, "An apple a day keeps the doctor away" is now backed by science. Research by Cornell University, the Cancer Research Center of Hawaii and the National Cancer Institute suggests that due to the nutrient content of Vitamin C, phytochemicals, flavanoids, antioxidiants and pectin, apples may reduce the risk of cancer by preventing DNA damage. Of all of the nutrient benefits of apples, I recommend them because of the pectin content. Pectin binds with toxins and heavy metals to remove them from the body. Other fruits that contain pectin are; blackberries, gooseberries, crab apples, cranberries, grapes, medlars, plums and quince. Any citrus fruit peel is also high in pectin. Fruits that are low in pectin are; apricots, blueberries, cherries, peaches, pears, raspberries, rhubarb, strawberries. Eating a whole apple is more nutritious that drinking an equal portion of apple juice since the fiber, vitamins and minerals may be processed out of the juices. In addition to their nutrient value, apples are an excellent source of dietary fiber with one medium size apple containing approximately thirteen percent of the recommended daily value. My favorite apple, hands down is the Fuji. I was introduced to the Fuji while living in Asia. The Fuji apple has exceptional firmness and juice and has a comparatively greater shelf life without refrigeration than other apples and can last up to 5 months without losing all of its nutrient value in the refrigerator. It originated in Japan in the 1930's and was introduced into the United States in the late 1980's.

Q:

Is there a natural remedy for bee stings?

A:

I never go anywhere in the summer months without an onion. A slice of onion on a yellow jacket, wasp, or bee sting, ant bite or scorpion bite works fantastic! Immediately the milky juice of the onion helps extract the poisons and reduce the swelling. And I bet you are wondering-white or yellow onion? Yellow onions are a bit stronger that the sweeter white onion, so pack a yellow one with you!

Q:

I recently had my homocysteine levels tested and found they were a bit elevated. Can you please tell me if there is a way that I can reduce these levels through diet? Also, I had been taking aspirin but developed gastric bleeding and had to stop so I am wondering if there is something natural that I can take in its place.

A:

First let me explain what homocysteine is for those that are unfamiliar with this term. Homocysteine is a body substance that helps manufacture proteins and assist with cellular metabolism. It is a harmless amino acid, but in excess, it can cause blood platelets to clump together and vascular walls to break down, which can lead to atherosclerosis and coronary artery disease. Research linking heart disease to elevated plasma levels of homocysteine began as early as 1969, when Dr. Kilmer McCully, a Harvard pathologist, found rare cases of severe atherosclerosis in children with very high homocysteine levels. Some factors that can contribute to high homocysteine levels are: Eating too much protein (because it converts a naturally containing amino acid methionine to homocysteine), Caffeine, Vitamin D deficiency, Smoking, Aging, Thyroid hormone deficiency, and some prescription drugs that deplete Vitamin B levels in the system. Four simple suggestions that can help re-balance your homocysteine levels are: Supplementation with a whole food Vitamin B complex, Garlic-which helps aortic elasticity, Ginger- which can take the place of aspirin since it inhibits a specific enzyme that makes the blood prone to stickiness just like aspirin but without the side effects, and red wine. Yes, red wine since it contains resveratrol which naturally has anticoagulant properties. As I always suggest, be sure to consult with your physician before starting any new program regarding diet to be sure there will be no complications with any medications that you are currently taking. And if your physician agrees-Cheers!

Q:

Can you please tell me what happens to your body when you quit smoking?

A:

Twenty minutes after you put that final cigarette out-your blood pressure drops to normal. Eight hours after -the carbon monoxide level in your blood drops to normal. Twenty four hours after- your chance of heart attack decreases. Forty eight after-nerve endings start re-growing, enhancing your smell again. Two weeks to three months after-circulation improves. One to nine months later-coughing, sinus congestion and shortness of breath decreases. Cilia regrows in your lungs. One year after- your risk of heart disease is cut in half. Five years after-lung cancer risk decreases by half, stroke risk is reduced, risk of throat, mouth and esophagus cancer is reduced by half of a smoker. Ten years after-precancerous cells are replaced and cancer risk continues to decline. Fifteen years after-coronary heart disease risk is that of a non smoker. Thanks to The American Cancer Society and the Center for Disease Control for help with this one!

Q:

I hope you can answer some egg questions for me. Do brown eggs have a higher nutritional value than white eggs? Can you look at an egg and tell if it is fresh? Is there a special secret to keeping the yolk in the middle of the egg when boiling for making deviled eggs? And, I accidently put some boiled eggs in with my fresh eggs-any way I can tell which ones were boiled?

A:

Calorie for calorie, protein for protein, fat for fat, brown eggs are equal to white eggs based on nutritional values! You can easily tell how fresh an egg is by the shell-fresh eggs have shells that are rough and chalky and old eggs have shells that are smooth and shiny! When cooking eggs for making deviled eggs, and to have that perfect deviled egg look, simply stir the water occasionally while they are cooking. Oops, put the boiled eggs in with the raw eggs- no problem. Just spin the egg (carefully, of course), and observe the spin. If it wobbles, it is raw and if it spins evenly it is hard boiled! Here are a few other facts about cackleberries that you may enjoy! It is best to store eggs with the tapered end down and the larger end upright as that maximizes the distance between the yolk and the air pocket, which may contain bacteria! Eggs should never be boiled longer than twelve minutes-cooking them longer results in a chemical change within the egg. The sulfur in the egg combines with the iron in the yolk which forms the harmless chemical ferrous sulfide. And about the producers-the average hen produces about two hundred and twenty five eggs a year, which converts to about three thousand eggs in a lifetime since they start laying eggs about five months after they are hatched! And now you know a little more about the wonderful egg!

Q:

I know you dislike the consumption of colas. I can understand the diet colas but what is so bad about regular colas?

A:

Did you know....A cola will dissolve a steak in two days! A cola will loosen a rusted bolt if soaked for ten minutes! A cola is great for cleaning toilets! Have rust on your bumper-pour a little cola on it! A cola will dissolve a nail in four days thanks to its phosphoric acid! Colas are used to clean truck engines! And last, did you know that transporters carrying cola syrup are required to display the hazardous placard that states: "Highly Corrosive Materials". So **Please**-Pass me the water!

Q:

I recently found myself in a mad dash to our TV room to catch a story on the television about the toxicity of phthalates and the dangers to pregnant women. I just caught the end of the story and was wondering if you have any information regarding phthalates. Since I am pregnant, I now have some concerns. I am eating healthy and have changed my lifestyle but I am not familiar with whatever these phthalates are and how I am exposed to them. Thank you!

A:

Phthalates (pronounced tha-lates) are plasticizer chemicals found in plastic and other materials used primarily to make the product soft and flexible. An astounding billion pounds are produced per year worldwide! Recently, laboratory studies at the US Environmental Protection Agency, has turned attention to low dose toxicity of phthalates during crucial windows of fetal development. The study, led by scientist Earl Gray, revealed that male reproductive development is acutely sensitive to phthalates. In another study, conducted by Dr. John Bucher, Associate Director of the US Department of Health and Human Services, Dr Bucher states it has been known since the late 1990's that certain phthalates specifically effect development of the male reproductive system during fetal development. While more studies are being conducted, some companies have already announced phase out polices regarding the use of phthalates. The following are a few of the many products that can contain phthalates; printing inks, paints, sealants, lubricants, pvc, lacquers, children's toys, emulsifying agents, personal care products, medical devices, nail polish, shower curtains, window shades, pencil erasers and some plastic food packaging. Additional intentional uses of phthalates include oily substances in perfumes, additives to hairsprays, lubricants and wood finishes. That new car smell, which becomes intense after the vehicle sits in the hot sun for a few hours, is partially the odor of phthalates volatilizing from a hot plastic dashboard. Once the car cools, phthalates condense out of the inside air of the vehicle to form the oily coating on the inside of the windshield.

Q:

I have changed by diet dramatically and have developed a taste for asparagus. Why are they so expensive compared to other vegetables?

A:

While asparagus is a member of the lily family which includes leeks, garlic and onions, asparagus are expensive because they have to be harvested by hand. Asparagus have many health benefits including the fact that it is one of the few vegetables that has the proper ratio of calcium and magnesium of 2:1. Asparagus is also a very alkaline vegetable which is why it is highly recommended for cancer patients.

Q:

I am a cancer survivor and I take green food supplements every day that contains barley grass, alfalfa and wheat grass. Can you please the share benefits of each of these grasses?

A:

Green grasses have the extraordinary ability to transform inanimate elements from soil, water, and sunlight into living cells with energy. Grasses contain all of the known minerals and trace minerals, vitamins and hundreds of enzymes. The greatest benefit is the small molecular proteins and chorophyllins in grasses that are absorbed directly through our cell membranes. Alfalfa is a legume while barley and wheat are cereal grasses. Alfalfa pulls up earth minerals from roots as deep as one hundred and fifty feet and contains high levels of chlorophyll. Alfalfa contains vitamin A, D, E, K, and B as well as silicon, phosphorous, iron, potassium, magnesium and many other trace elements. Alfalfa also has eight known enzymes that promote chemical reactions that enable food to be assimilated properly within the body. Barley grass has eleven times more calcium than cow's milk, five times more iron than spinach, and seven times more vitamin C and bioflavoids than orange juice (without the sugar). Barley grass is an ideal aniti-inflammatory for healing gastrointestinal ulcers, hemorrhoids and pancreatic functions. Wheat grass is a vegetable therefore it does not contain gluten since the leaf is harvested before the seed develops. Fifteen pounds of fresh wheat grass has the nutritional value of three hundred and fifty pounds of vegetables with all of the enzyme activity. As with all the green grasses, it ability to provide protection from carcinogens comes from chlorophyll's capacity to strengthen cells, detoxify the liver and blood, and biochemically neutralize pollutants. The blend of these three grasses contributes greatly to the alkaline reserves and in helping to keep acid/alkaline balance in the body neutral which is very important if you are a cancer survivor.

Q:

I recently connected with a friend and he told me he was a pesco vegetarian. I always thought a vegetarian was someone that just did not eat meat so now I wonder what types of vegetarians are there?

A:

Here is a sampling; Vegan: excludes all animal derived foods. Ovo vegetarian: eats eggs, but no other animal products. Semi vegetarian: eat poultry, fish, eggs, and diary but no red meats or pork. Lacto ovo vegetarian: eats eggs and diary foods, but no animal food that has "eyes" and finally your Pesco vegetarian: eats fish, eggs, and diary foods, but no poultry, red meats or pork. If I have missed one, I apologize and ask that you please contact me and share with me your style.

Q:

I am a diabetic and was told how I should avoid potatoes since they are a high glycemic index food. Someone told me I should try sunchokes. Can you please tell me about sunchokes?

A:

Sunchoke is also known as Jerusalem artichoke, although it is not an artichoke and it is not from Jerusalem. Sunchoke is actually a tuber that looks like ginger root, has a potato like texture and is highly recommended as a potato substitute for diabetics. Because of the high inulin content, sunchoke has a very low glycemic index. The glycemic index, simply stated, is the rate at which your body converts food to sugar. Lower glycemic index foods are usually more nutritious and healthier for your system. Sunchoke can be eaten raw, roasted, boiled, baked, and my least favorite-fried, or cooked and like many root vegetables, it is a good source of potassium, fiber, niacin and some of the B vitamins.

Q:

I am a tea drinker and enjoy a cup of hot tea daily. Can you please tell me the difference between green tea, oolong tea and black tea and is one better than the other?

A:

All black, green and Oolong teas come from one plant, *thea sinensis*, an incredibly productive shrub that grows from the Mediterranean to the tropics. The tea leaves can be continuously harvested every six to fourteen days for up to fifty years. All teas are defined by the way the leaves are actually processed. With green tea, the tender leaves are picked, rolled, steamed, crushed, and dried with hot air but never fermented. Oolong teas are semi-fermented and black tea is fermented for three hours and need to be scented to reduce bitterness. While both the green and black teas contain enzymes that promote digestion, green tea, by far, contains the most health benefits. Green tea contains twice as much vitamin C, twice the amount of bioflavonoids, and six times the antioxidant properties of black tea. Green tea contains over two hundred different catechin polyphenols that comprise up to thirty five percent of green tea. In addition, green tea is a vasodilator and smooth muscle relaxer for bronchial dilation against asthma. According to Dr. John Weisburger, researcher at the Institute for Cancer Prevention, laboratory test show that green tea may help boost metabolism to aid weight loss, block allergic response, slow the growth of tumors, protect bones, fight bad breath, is a heart health protector, improves skin, protect against Parkinson's disease and can even delay the onset of diabetes. If you are a tea drinker, do not add milk to green tea. Milk inhibits the absorption of the protective polyphenols. Removing the caffeine naturally through a water process, does not affect the benefits of the polyphenols and bioflavonoids. Now you know that black, oolong or green tea refers to the tea leaf process. Did you know that Darjeeling, Earl Gray or Ceylon refer to the country or region where the tea is grown and names like, pekoe, orange pekoe refer to the leaf size?

Q:

Excess salt in a person's diet was recently in the news with questions about if the government should be involved. The government became involved long ago when it was decided that people were not getting enough iodide. I do not add table salt to my meals so I wonder if I get the iodide that I need. Also, is sea salt the best salt to use?

A:

First, a quick bit of salt history. The word salary comes from the Latin word for salt, a connection that dates back to the time when Roman soldiers were paid with salt. Hence the phrase evolved of people saying as they headed to work; " I'm off to the salt mine". Salt is one of the essential elements of life. However, the human body cannot produce salt, therefore we have to take it from an external source. Most of the salt we get comes from refined table salt. The problem is that the human body does not know how to handle processed salt, which is refined table salt. While the debate continues about salt, what we know for a fact is that the body needs sodium and potassium, the electrolytes that the body uses to control water levels in the blood and tissues. An excess or deficiency of EITHER of these ions can be life threatening. If we eat a diet largely based on natural foods, we need some sodium. Vegetables and fruits, on the other hand, provide us with the potassium that the body needs, although the balance of both sodium and potassium are both necessary. Iodine is the elemental (basic) name of the mineral. When it is combined with any thing else, it becomes iodide. Therefore, iodide is a form of iodine that is preferentially taken up by the thyroid gland (the reason manufacturers began adding iodine to salt in the 1920's was to prevent goiters-an enlarged thyroid gland caused by an iodine deficiency). Sea salt contains iodide, actually 8.76 PPM (parts per millions) and over seventy other minerals. Because of these extra minerals, sea salt brings a more subtle, complex flavor to the foods it is used to season and is not as "salty" as refined table salt. While sea salt and table salt are both sodium chloride, sea salt may contain less iodine so it is important to select a sea salt that is ionized. If you use a sea salt that is not ionized, you can add more seafood to your diet since it is a natural source of iodine as well as kelp powder. As a note, the sodium chloride used in processed foods is NOT iodized. A closing factoid: Higher sodium intake increases your calcium needs because as sodium intake climbs, more calcium is lost in the urine.

Q:

I eat very healthy and take a whole food multi vitamin every day. My friends are always asking me why I take the vitamins thinking that because I eat healthy I do not need daily supplements. Some of my friends claim that they can't take vitamins because the vitamins bother their stomach. For my friends and all others that read your column, can you please help me explain this one?

A:

Three important points as to why we need to take vitamins revolve around our food. First, our soil is depleted of minerals, causing our food to be deficient, second, our modern processing methods destroys nutrients (i.e. canned foods are all cooked in the cans), and third, we overcook our food destroying what few nutrients are left after the processing. A USDA (United States Department of Agriculture) survey of 21,500 people found that ***not one single person*** consumed 100% of the U. S. RDA (recommended daily allowance) from the foods they ate. Healthy, live food is essential to our cells since every one hundred days our red bloods cells are replaced, every five to ten days the lining of our gastrointestinal tract is replaced with new cells and every thirty days our skin is replaced with new cells, just to name a few. In some areas of our bodies, the process is even faster. A corneal abrasion, for example, only takes two days to heal according to Don Colbert, M.D. As your cells die and are being replaced, the new cells are totally dependent on what building materials are available. While supplements are not a substitute for eating healthy foods, taking whole food supplements daily can be beneficial to the body. However, many vitamins have synthetics added to increase potency, or to standardize the amount in a capsule or batch. Synthetic vitamins are made from coal tar derivatives, and, in addition, a salt form is added to increase stability of the nutrient. The following terms listed in the ingredients help identify if a supplement is synthetic; acetate, bitartrate, chloride, gluconate, hydrochloride, nitrate or succinate. Synthetic substances may cause reactions to chemically susceptible individuals while the same individual can easily tolerate naturally derived, whole food supplements without any problems. Natural or whole food supplements contain the total complex family of micro-nutrients just as they are found in nature. These micronutrients are indispensable for proper vitamin absorption and maximum utilization-something synthetic vitamins lack. And for those individuals that have a difficult time taking supplements, it may be because many supplements contain gluten which can cause stomach discomfort-especially to those individuals that have been diagnosed with Celiac disease.

Q:

I have been diagnosed with breast cancer and in some of the literature I was given, it says I should avoid products that contain soy. Now that I am a diligent label reader, I am amazed at how many products contain soy isoflavones. Can you explain what isoflavones are and why they can be dangerous ?

A:

Americans are eating more soy products than ever before and in fact now consume more than the Japanese and Chinese do. While the Asian practice of fermenting soybeans and eating soy in the form of curds called tofu can be healthy, Asians consume soy in very small amounts, as a condiment, rather than a food replacement for animal proteins as is the common practice in the United States. The soybean itself is a notably inauspicious staple food; it contains a whole assortment of "antinutrients", which are compounds that actually block the body's absorption of vitamins and minerals, interfere with the hormonal system, and prevent the body from breaking down the proteins in the soy itself. Soy isoflavones, found in most soy products, are compounds that resemble, and in fact, bind to human estrogen receptors. It is unclear whether these so called phytoestrogens actually behave like estrogens or fool the body into thinking they are estrogen. Because they may have an effect on the growth of certain cancers, the symptoms of menopause and the function of the endocrine system, the FDA, Food and Drug Administration, has declined to grant GRAS (Generally Regarded As Safe) status to soy isoflavones for use as food additives although some soy products do have the GRAS rating.

Q:

I try to eat healthy because I know that everything you eat is processed through the liver. What are some of the most important functions of the liver and what foods are best for the liver?

A:

The liver performs over five hundred functions in the human body. While all the functions are important, it is impossible to list them all so here is a list of some of the more important duties;

- Metabolize proteins, fats, and carbohydrates
- Stores vitamins, minerals and sugar
- Filters the blood and helps remove toxins
- Breaks down and eliminates excess hormones
- Helps maintain electrolyte balance and water balance

- Helps to assimilate and store fat soluble vitamins, A, D, E, K
- Removes damaged red blood cells
- Provides blood clotting factors
- Removes ammonia, a toxic by-product of animal protein metabolism, from the body
- Breaks down hormones after they have done their function, i.e. if the liver does not break down insulin fast enough, hypoglycemia results because the circulating insulin continues to lower blood sugar.

The top ten foods that benefit the liver the most are apples, artichoke, dandelion, beets, garlic, lemon (in hot water), cabbage, broccoli, strawberries and onions (in this order).

Q:

I keep hearing and reading about Vitamin D and its importance. I would appreciate it if you could answer the following questions: how much do we need daily, what are the benefits of Vitamin D, and what are the best food sources of Vitamin D?

A:

Studies continue to flood the news about the benefits of vitamin D. While these studies have indicated it is essential for the heart, bones and almost everything in between. Vitamin D also protects against disease such as cancer and diabetes. Current dietary guidelines recommends four hundred IU of vitamin D daily, however, according to Dr. Stephen Sinatra, Cardiologist, his recommendation is 2,000-5,000 IU a day. Dr. Sinatra states that because the average person doesn't spend enough time in the sunlight to produce serum D levels linked to better health, supplementation is more important than ever. According to Mayo Clinic, the major biological function of vitamin D is to maintain normal blood levels of calcium and phosphorous. Recent research also suggests that vitamin D may provide protection from osteoporosis, high blood pressure, cancer and several autoimmune diseases. While vitamin D intake is important, if you suffer from adenoma of the parathyroid gland, granulomatous diseases, lymphoma, sarcoidosis, and tuberculosis, these conditions may cause your body to produce too much vitamin D, increasing your risk of developing an elevated calcium level. As always, I recommend you talk with your physician before starting a vitamin D supplementation program or, for that matter, any supplements. The best food sources of vitamin D is salmon (cooked-NOT farm raised) contains 360 IU for a 3 ½ oz. serving, Mackerel (cooked-NOT farm raised) has 345 IU for a 3 1/2 oz. serving and sardines, canned in oil & drained, contains 270 IU for 3 ½ oz. serving. Egg has 25 IU per egg and cod liver oil tops the chart with 450 IU for 1 teaspoon.

Q:

You recently mentioned in your column a few comments about onions. I would appreciate if you could elaborate a bit more about onions. You have previously listed nuts from in order of nutrient value, so I am wondering if there is one onion variety that is better than another?

A:

Onions do have a ranking order with some being better than others based on their antioxidant level. If you can't remember the names, just remember that the sweeter or milder tasting the onion is, the *fewer* antioxidiants it contains. The order, starting with number one;Shallots (which are related to onions), Western White, Western Yellow, Imperial Valley Sweet, Northern Red and Vidalia. It is best to not store onions in the fridge, or near potatoes. Potatoes give off moisture and a gas that causes onions to spoil faster. If you are going to eat onions raw, be sure to wash them thoroughly since they grow underground they can harbor nasty bacteria. Here are a few home uses for onions that you may find interesting! Onion is great for bee stings and removing rust from knife blades. Rub onion on your skin for repelling mosquitoes and biting insects! It worked great for us in Africa!

Q:

I am a coffee drinker and really enjoy my coffee each morning and afternoon. I was recently diagnosed with a mild heart condition and my doctor suggested that I avoid caffeine and recommended that I switch to decaffeinated. When I look at labels, I see that there are decaffeinated and *naturally* decaffeinated teas and coffees. Is there a difference and if so can you please explain?

A:

Yes, there is a difference between decaffeinated and naturally decaffeinated coffee and tea. Coffee can be decaffeinated using one of several methods. One process of decaffeinating is a chemical process, using solvents such as formaldehyde, which absorb the caffeine from the bean to remove it. Another process of decaffeination uses water to remove the caffeine by soaking the beans prior to roasting. Water decaffeination is considered to be the healthiest process and is referred to as *Naturally* decaffeinated. A variant of the water method is the carbon dioxide method. In this process the beans are steamed and then soaked in carbonated water. The water is then drained through a charcoal filter. There is one additional process that soaks green coffee beans in a water and coffee solution to remove caffeine. Most companies that produce decaffeinated coffees are happy to share their information regarding the process of decaffeination they use. It is important to know that decaffeinated coffee is not one hundred percent caffeine free but that the caffeine is reduced by about ninety seven percent. In order for a coffee product to be labeled decaffeinated, it must have at least ninety seven percent of its caffeine removed.

Q:

What are your dietary recommendations for someone with Lupus?

A:

Lupus most often refers to a condition that affects many systems of the body, including skin, joints, and kidney. Lupus is a classic example of an autoimmune-type disease in which the body's immune system attacks connective tissue, causing pain and inflammation and affects women nine times more than men. An internal acidic environment promotes pain and inflammation so it is important to eat as many raw vegetables and citrus fruits to help return the body to an alkaline state. These foods are also high in fiber which can help relieve digestive problems and high in antioxidants which counteract inflammation. Onions, garlic, asparagus, flaxseeds and wheat germ are excellent. Avoid saturated fats, hydrogenated fats, partially hydrogenated fats, fried and greasy foods. It is best to eliminate sugar, alcohol, caffeine and canned sodas. These products can damage the immune system and leave you even more susceptible to infection and illness.

Q:

If there is a spot of mold on a slice of bread, is it safe to break off that spot and eat the bread?

A:

I would strongly recommend not eating the bread. When mold grows on soft food like bread, just removing the visible mold spot does not remove all of the spores. Mold actually consists of root threads that invade the food it lands on, with a stalk rising above the food and spores forming on the end of those stalks. The root threads can grow deep into the food and have poisonous substances around the threads. If you ingest any part, on or around the mold spores, it could very likely cause gastrointestinal problems, such as diarrhea. If you spot mold on lunch meats, bacon, hot dogs, cottage cheese, cream cheese, yogurts, jams, jellies, peanut butter, leftovers, bread, and soft produce such as cucumbers peaches and tomatoes, I would recommend discarding the food to prevent a possible gastrointestinal event. However, you can safely excise a moldy area from firm foods such as hard cheese. If you do cut this moldy area out, be sure to include at least a one half inch margin of safety all around the mold. If there is mold on hard salami or dry-cured ham, the mold can be scrubbed away and the food safely eaten. Molds on firm fruit and vegetables such as cabbage, bell peppers and carrots, can be cut away with one inch of surrounding flesh and safely eaten.

Q:

My nonfat yogurt lists 5 milligrams of cholesterol. How can a food have cholesterol but no fat? Also, I do enjoy my beer and if it does not contain any fat or cholesterol where do the calories come from?

A:

It is possible for a food to have no fat and some cholesterol but it is not very common. Foods that have no fat, including most grains, vegetables and fruits, generally do not contain cholesterol either. Nonfat yogurt and skim milk are among the few exceptions. Many more foods, especially those that contain vegetable oils, have fat but no cholesterol. The reason is because cholesterol is found only in animal products such as meat, eggs, milk, and cheese. That is why it is no trick for a bag of potato chips or a tub of margarine to declare "no cholesterol". As for your second question, the calories in beer come from alcohol, carbohydrates, and a minuscule amount of protein.

Q:

I have thrown out my microwave for safety reasons and was wondering how a convection oven works compared to a microwave?

A:

The standard oven and the convection oven, work similar to each other. The notable difference in the convection oven is that it has a fan that increases the distribution of the heat molecules providing heat to all areas more evenly and faster. Because of the fan and the efficiency of the heat circulation, a lower temperature is usually required, thereby conserving energy. Meats do very well cooked in a convection oven, and because of the lower heat, the meat tends to be juicer! Microwaves, on the other hand, penetrate and are absorbed by food products and liquids. The energy penetrates the food and its power is gradually absorbed, or lost, to each layer of molecules. The rate of energy loss and depth of penetration vary depending on the food. Hence, microwaved food is quite often found cold in the center. The Journal of the Science of Food and Agriculture has stated that research shows that microwaving food does cause a significant decrease in the nutritive value of food.

Q:

I know how important drinking water is but I would like to know if there are guidelines for when it is best to drink water? Is there a simple rule of thumb for how much water we should drink daily?

A:

Here are a few simple suggestions according to Dr. F. Batmanghelidj, M.D. author of *You're Not Sick You're Thirsty.*

- Water should be consumed no more than thirty minutes before meals with a squeeze of lemon or lime in the water. This prepares the digestive tract and is especially important for individuals with gastritis, heartburn, peptic ulcer, colitis and indigestion.
- Water should be taken approximately two hours after a meal to complete the process of digestion and correct the dehydration cause by the food breakdown.
- Water should be taken first thing in the morning to correct dehydration-the result of the long hours of sleep.
- Water should be taken before exercising to have it available for creating sweat.
- Do not wait to drink water. When you are thirsty-you are probably already dehydrated.

I recommend that we consume one half of our body weight in ounces of water daily. To help you figure this out-If you weigh one hundred and twenty pounds that would convert to sixty ounces of water daily. This is in addition to any other beverages you consume during the course of a day. Remember the number one cause of daytime fatigue is dehydration!

Q:

I have a quick question. I was reading through some recipes and came across one that called for Squab! Can you please tell me what SQUAB is? I am writing this letter because I am too old to learn about computers and research this myself. Thank you for your help.

A:

Squab is a "mini pigeon" that is no more than one month old. Squab has been bred for centuries dating back to early Asian and Arabic cultures. According to the Squab Producers of California, careful breeding and a specially formulated diet of natural high proteins and whole grains produces meatier birds. For this reason, the meat of a Squab is distinctly unlike domestic poultry or wild game birds. Squab also possess a characteristic which allows them to retain more moisture during the cooking process than other poultry and is known to be one of the easily digestible of all meats. Squab are usually sold frozen, will store frozen for about six months, and will not weigh more than one pound. Look for birds with pale skin and the plumper-the better.

Q:

I am overly sensitive to sodium and have to watch my intake very carefully! I do love to cook and wonder if you can tell me if there are any spices that are sodium free!

A:

The average person consumes about four thousand, five hundred mg. of salt daily which converts to about two teaspoons while the body only requires two hundred mg. daily which converts to about one quarter of a teaspoon daily. Many spices do contain sodium as a part of their general make-up, but the following are some spices and flavorings that are sodium free; Allspice, Caraway seeds, Garlic, Mace, Mustard powder, Parsley, Rosemary, Sesame seed, Vanilla Extract, Almond Extract, Cinnamon, Ginger, Maple Extract, Nutmeg, Pepper, Peppermint, Thyme, Walnut Extract, Bay Leaves, Curry Powder, Lemon Extract, Marjoram, Paprika, Pimento, Extract of Sage, Turmeric and Vinegar.

Q:

Can you please explain the difference between pure, cold pressed, extra virgin and virgin olive oil. Also, is there a particular reason why olive oil is always in a glass container?

A:

PURE olive oil indicates that there is only one variety of oil, not a blend, and can be heated safely. COLD PRESSED is a process in which non-preheated oil seeds are pressed only once, with no additional heat and at the lowest temperature possible, never exceeding 50 degrees, to extract the oil. This type of pressing preserves the nutritional properties of the oil. EXTRA VIRGIN applies to olive oil only. It means that it is the best quality olive oil with the lowest oleic acidity which is less the .08%. Extra virgin olive oil is not designed to be heated. VIRGIN OLIVE OIL is the equivalent of first cold pressed and can be used for all varieties of oil. Virgin also refers to second quality and the oleic acidity of virgin olive oil is 1.5%. Because of the high quality of olive oil, the optimum storage containers are ceramic jars, glass bottles (dark bottles are even better) and tin cans since air and light are enemies of olive oil.

Q:

Are products that are wheat free also gluten free? Also, are there flours that are wheat free and gluten free?

A:

For your first question, not necessarily! Gluten free products are safe for someone with Celiac disease, but gluten free does not always mean wheat free unless the label specifically states the product is wheat free. Wheat free means there are no wheat flour ingredients in a food and are helpful to those who have wheat allergies. Gluten is a component of many grains including wheat, barley and rye, so the term gluten free food is a much more restrictive food in that it does not contain any of these derivatives. While wheat is one of the most common food allergens, Gluten is toxic to the small intestine and damages it, preventing nutrients from being absorbed into the body. And for your second question, the following are wheat **and** gluten free flours; Amaranth flour, Soy flour, Arrowroot flour, Brown/White rice flour, Buckwheat flour, Chickpea flour, Maize flour, Millet flour, Quinoa (keen-wa) flour, Sorghum flour and Teff flour.

Q:

Is it true that food colorants cochineal and carmine are made from ground beetles? Are there other names for the same type of coloring? Is this toxic to humans?

A:

Cochineal and carmine, also known as carminic acid, are derived from the crushed carcasses of the female dactylopius coccus, a beetle that inhabits a type of cactus in Central and South America. These colorants are used today to color candies, fruit juices, gelatins, jams, yogurts, milk, sausage, marinades, sauces, cola drinks, popsicles, cosmetics and shampoos. While some food labels may list the coloring as cochineal or carmine, these ingredients are also known as red #4, natural red, E120, carminic acid and crimson lake so it is important to know all of these colorings. Some individuals are sensitive to food colorings, natural or otherwise, so it is important to be diligent in reading food labels since these color additives may cause asthma, upper respiratory distress or even anaphyalactic shock. It takes 155,000 beetles to make about two pounds of cochineal.

Q:

I cook a lot with butter and wonder if it makes a difference if it is salted or unsalted. Also, what causes butter to burn so quickly? Is there anything I can do to stop the scorching?

A:

If you purchase the "salted" butter, it can contain anywhere from 1.5% to 1.3% salt content. This can play havoc with certain recipes unless you are aware of the actual salt content of a particular butter and how the level of salt in that butter will react with your recipe. It is usually easier to use "unsalted" butter and add your sea salt or lite salt. When butter is heated, the protein goes through a change, and causes the butter to burn and scorch easily. A small amount of pure olive oil (NOT extra virgin oil since that type of oil is not to be heated) will slow the process down. If clarified butter is used, butter in which the protein has been removed, you can fry or sauté with it and it will last for a longer period of time than standard butter. However, clarified butter will not give your foods that real, rich butter flavor. An interesting note about butter-if you are heating milk up in a pot, spread a very thin layer of unsalted butter on the bottom of the pot to prevent the milk from sticking. If you use salted butter-this will not work!

Q:

Can you please me about hemp milk. I cannot tolerate regular milk and do not care for soy milk, so I am wondering if this is a healthier substitute.

A:

Hemp milk is made from hemp seeds that are soaked and ground into water, yielding a creamy nutty tasting beverage. An eight ounce serving of hemp milk, depending on brand, can contain up to 900 mg. of Omega 3 fatty acids, 2800 mg. of Omega 6 fatty acids, all ten of the essential amino acids, four grams of digestive proteins, and forty six percent of the recommended daily allowance of calcium. Hemp milk also contains potassium, phosphorous, riboflavin, vitamin A, vitamin E, vitamin B12, vitamin D, folic acid, magnesium, iron and zinc. Plain organic hemp milk contains no cholesterol, no trans fats and is completely free of soy and gluten. Hemp protein, from which the milk is made, does not contain high levels of enzyme inhibitors, phytates, which can interfere with the proper assimilation of essential minerals or oligosaccharides, which can cause flatulence (gas) and stomach distress.

Q:

This may be a dumb question but could you please tell me what some of the healthiest vegetables would be? What makes some vegetables healthier than others?

A:

No question is ever a dumb question so thank you for asking! Here is a list of the top twenty vegetables based on their nutrient levels of ten of the most important nutrients. The ten nutrients these vegetables include are protein, iron, calcium, niacin, vitamin a, vitamin C, potassium, phosphorus, thiamin and riboflavin. In descending order, here are the best; Collard Greens, Lima Beans, Peas, Spinach, Sweet Potato, Turnip Greens, Winter Squash, Broccoli, Kale, Brussels Sprouts, Mustard Greens, Swiss Chard, Parsley, Tomatoes (NOT genetically modified), Corn (NOT genetically modified), Beet Greens, Pumpkin, Okra, Potatoes and Carrots.

Q:

I am noticing more articles about the dangers of drinking out of Styrofoam? What makes it so dangerous? It scares me a bit since I asked my grandmother if she ever drank out of Styrofoam and she said all she ever drank was water out of a glass! Can you help clear the air?

A:

First, let me explain, that what we refer to as Styrofoam, should really be referred to as a polystyrene. Styrofoam is a trademark material made by the Dow Chemical Company, and they do not make cups, plates, egg trays or other types of food packaging. Now, to your question; each time you drink or eat out of a "polystyrene" container, the basic chemical component, styrene, has the potential to leach into your food or beverage and then into you. The migration of styrene from a polystyrene cup into the food or beverage it contains has been observed to be as high a 0.025% for a single use. Styrene migration has been shown to be partially dependent on the fat content of the food in the polystyrene cup or container. In other words, the higher the fat content, the more styrene will be pulled out of the styrene container. Styrene also appears to migrate more quickly when a beverage poured into a styrene container is hot. Studies suggest that styrene mimics estrogen in the body and can possibly disrupt normal hormone functions. The International Agency for Research on Cancer lists styrene as a possible human carcinogen. My recommendation is to use as much glass, lead-free ceramic, stainless steel (not aluminum) and paper to consume food and beverage products out of.

Q:

As a diabetic, I am very leery of using any artificial sweetener. Is there anything on the market that is safe and natural and has a low glycemic index? My friends have told me about Xylitol, but I need a bit more information before I try it!

A:

The Food and Drug Administration confirmed in 1986 that Xylitol is a safe sweetener. Xylitol is not actually a sugar, but a sugar alcohol and was discovered by German and French chemists in the late 19th century. During World War II, there was a shortage of sugar and researchers were forced to look at alternative sweeteners. It was during this period when Finnish researchers re-discovered xylitol, the low calorie sugar alcohol that came from birch tree bark(you do not want that made from corn). It has since been used for decades around the world as a sweetener for diabetics because of xylitol's insulin dependent nature (it metabolizes in the body without using insulin). What makes xylitol safe is that it is considered a five carbon sugar, which means it is antimicrobial, preventing the growth of bacteria. All other forms of sugar are six carbon sugars which feeds dangerous bacteria and fungi. While sugar is acid forming, xylitol is alkaline enhancing. An interesting fact is that xylitol is produced naturally in our bodies, in fact, we make up to fifteen grams daily during normal metabolism. While research indicates that xylitol can sicken or even be fatal to dogs, do not let that worry you since chocolate, raisins, grapes, nuts, tomatoes and onions may also be problematic to your pooch!

Q:

I have a friend who has arthritis and he told me he eats very few nightshades and how much better his arthritis is. Can you please explain what nightshades are?

A:

Potatoes, tomatoes, sweet and hot peppers, and eggplant are classified as nightshade foods and are the most common out of about two thousand nightshade plants. A particular group of substances in these foods called alkaloids, can impact nerve-muscle function and digestion function in humans and may be able to compromise joint function. Because the amount of alkaloid is very low in nightshade foods when compared to other nightshade plants, health problems from nightshade foods may only occur in individuals who are especially sensitive to these alkaloid substances. Since cooking nightshade foods only lowers the alkaloid content by forty to fifty percent, sensitive individuals may want to avoid these foods altogether if they suffer from arthritis. If you suffer from arthritis, it is important to evaluate your diet and also consider eliminating gluten, dairy, moldy foods (i.e. aged cheese) and increase your water intake.

Q:

I have heart disease and was recently told my homocysteine levels are elevated. Can you please tell me how I can lower my homocysteine levels naturally and safely as to not to interfere with my medication.

A:

According to Mayo Clinic, a high homocysteine level may be associated with an increased risk of cardiovascular disease and is a risk factor for stroke. The New England Journal of Medicine (April 9, 1998) and The Journal of The American Medical Association (JAMA, December 18, 1996) published articles suggesting that vitamin supplements be used to lower homocysteine levels. High levels of homocysteine have been linked to lower levels of folic acid, vitamin B6, and vitamin B12. You may consider changing your diet to include more green, leafy vegetables that are high in folic acid like spinach, asparagus, and collard greens, which are exceptional sources that are also low in calories. Foods that are high in protein contain B6 and B12 like eggs, legumes (i.e. peas, beans, nuts), pork, chicken, meat, and fish. In addition to a healthier diet, if you take a whole food supplement of B6, B12 and folic acid, it is best to avoid synthetic supplements, so look for the supplement label to say ***whole food source***. The American Heart Association recommends taking four hundred mcg daily of folic acid. The Harvard School of Public Health recommends 1.3 to 1.7 mg. of vitamin B6 daily and 2.4 mcg. of vitamin B12 daily. And finally, stop smoking, avoid alcohol and eliminate caffeine.

Q:

I love trivia and was wondering if there was a chance you can share some food trivia?

A:

Did you know.....Lemons contain more sugar than strawberries? Catfish are the only animals that naturally have an ODD number of whiskers? Human saliva has a boiling point three times that of water? Intelligent people have more zinc and copper in their hair? Honey is the only food that will never spoil? An Ostrich egg takes four hours to boil? Cast iron skillets used to be the leading source of iron in the American diet? Each American eats an average of 51 pounds of chocolate a year! (and I do not eat any so someone is getting my share!)The FDA (Food and Drug Administration) allows 30 or more insect fragments and one or more rodent hairs in 100 grams of peanut butter! Apples-NOT CAFFEINE-are more efficient at waking you up in the morning! There are more nutrients in the cornflake package than there are in the corn flakes themselves! Rennet, a common substance used to culture milk and make cheese, is taken from the inner lining of the fourth stomach of a calf! And finally, according to a report issued by the Senate Committee on Nutrition and Human Needs, improving nutrition would cut the national health bill by approximately one-third.

Q:

Recently I ate some "healthy" ice cream and got a terrible case of brain freeze. Can you please explain what causes brain freeze?

A:

Brain freeze, referred to as sphenopalatine ganglineuralgia, is a reaction triggered when something very cold, in your case the ice cream, comes into contact with the roof of the mouth before you swallow. When something very cold, food or drink, touches the center of the palate, the cold temperature triggers nerves that control how much blood flows to the head. To heat up the brain again, the nerves respond by causing the blood vessels to swell which causes the headache pain. Even though this is referred to as "brain freeze", nothing is really happening in the brain-it is all in the blood vessels of the head. This reaction from cold food usually lasts a minute or two, although it seems to last much longer, and the headache usually goes away on its own. To eliminate developing "brain freeze" simply eating cold foods more slowly can help. You can also try warming that cold food or drink in the front of your mouth before swallowing.

Q:

I am a label reader but I cannot find anywhere on a label where the food originated from. I am a bit weary of consuming foods from foreign countries, especially China, after the tainted food scare in 2008. Am I missing something on the label?

A:

The bar code on the product indicates the country of origin. The first two, or in some cases the first three digits, listed on a product are referred to as the "Flag" and those numbers indicate in what country the bar code was issued. If the bar code on a product begins with 690-695, the product was made in China. Some countries bar codes only have two numbers like the Unites States and Canada whose code is 00-13, Japan-49, UK-50, Switzerland-76 and Spain-84 to name a few. Other bar codes are Mexico-750, Taiwan-471, Singapore-888, Thailand-885 and Malaysia-955. Currently, the United States and Canada use UPC bar codes as their standard, whereas the rest of the world uses EAN. Since January 1, 2005 all retail scanning systems in the USA must be able to accept the EAN symbol as well as the standard UPC. For a more detailed list of bar codes, please visit my web site, www. docphyl.com. If you do not find a particular code listed, please contact me. Thank you for reading your labels!

Q:

Not long ago I suffered a gout attack. I have changed my diet dramatically by eliminating purines but what else can I do to prevent another attack?

A:

Eliminating purines is very important since purines are organic compounds that contribute to uric acid formation. Be sure the list of purines you are eliminating includes the following; anchovies, asparagus, consummes and broths, herring, meat gravies, mushrooms, mussels, sardines, and sweet breads. In addition, it is important to eliminate the following: Meats-because they contain high levels of uric acid and that includes organ meats, Alcohol-because it increases the production of uric acid, Glycine- because this amino acid can be converted to uric acid more rapidly, rich foods such as cakes and pies, caffeine and refined sugars. The following foods needs to be consumed in moderation; cauliflower, dried beans, lentils, fish, eggs, oatmeal, peas, poultry, spinach and all yeast products. Drink plenty of water since fluid intake promotes the excretion of uric acid. Cherries, blueberries and strawberries neutralize uric acid, so it is important to include these fruits in your diet. Cherry juice is excellent. Flaxseeds are a highly concentrated source of essential fatty acids, the good "fats", that can help reduce inflammation. Take a whole food multi vitamin daily since a deficiency of pantothenic acid produces excessive amounts of uric acid and a vitamin E deficiency causes damage to the nuclei of cells that produce uric acid, causing more uric acid to form.

Q:

I recently purchased some Blackstrap molasses to use as a healthier sweetener. Can you please explain to me how molasses is made, and is there such a thing as Organic Molasses? Who consumes the most blackstrap molasses?

A:

Here are a few tidbits of info about Blackstrap Molasses that I would like to share: drop for drop, it contains more calcium than milk, more iron than beef, and more potassium that bananas. The word "molasses" is derived from the Portuguese word "melaco" which means "honey like" and is considered a natural sweetener. Blackstrap molasses is actually the concentrated byproduct syrup left over when the sugar's sucrose has been crystallized during the third boiling (dark molasses is the result of the second boiling). The largest producers of blackstrap molasses are India, Brazil, Taiwan, Thailand, the Philippines and the United States. There are three types of molasses, sulphured, unsulphured and blackstrap. Unsulphured molasses is the finest quality and blackstrap molasses made from organic sugar is now available. For a final bit of true trivia-in 1919 The Great Molasses Flood occurred when a molasses storage tank that held two million gallons of the viscous syrup burst in Boston. The molasses tsunami poured through a street in Boston at thirty five miles per hour creating a thirty foot tidal wave that killed twenty one people. And finally- the largest consumer of Blackstrap molasses??? Drum roll please-COWS! The majority of blackstrap molasses is manufactured for use in commercial cattle feed.

Q:

I love to cook with onions, but what is it about onions that make my eyes water, like I am crying, when I am cutting one up?

A:

A fresh onion, when cut, releases a gas called propanethiol-S into the air. When this gas reaches your eyes, it mixes with the water in the eye to form a weak acid. This acid irritates the eye and causes the tear producing glands to flood the eye with water in an attempt to flush away the irritant. These tears are what make it look like you are crying! For me, the simple solution is I whistle while I am cutting up onions-it works every time! How does that work you ask? The wind simply blows the gas away from your eyes! Warning-you will have everyone in your house peering around the corner wondering why you are so happy in the kitchen!

Q:

I recently traveled to Canada and noticed their food "pyramid" was actually a rainbow. Since you have traveled abroad so much, I was wondering if you know the shapes of other countries "pyramids"? Also, do you agree with the U.S. food pyramid?

A:

First off, I applaud your keen observation! Keep eating your carrots! While the United States uses the pyramid shape to illustrate how a healthful diet should be constructed, here are the food "pyramids" from around the world that I have observed. Israel uses a chalice, Japan arranges their food in the number 6 to represent the six food groups, Portugal, Germany, Norway and the United Kingdom put their food guides in the shape of a circle, Denmark uses a compass, Hungry uses a house, Mexico uses a plate, China and Korea use a pagoda, Thailand uses an inverted pyramid and the Philippines use a star. South Africa food graphic contains the least number of food groups and organizes food in a unique way-according to the food's function in the body. Group One contains "energy" foods like maize and grains, Group Two contains " body building foods" including chicken and beans and Group Three contains "protective foods" like fruits and vegetables. South America does not use a food pyramid. Most other countries have adopted the United States version. The food pyramid was designed to create a simple pictorial representation of dietary guidelines conveying relative amounts to eat from the various food groups. Unfortunately, the pyramid does not distinguish between whole grains and refined grains-a growing problem since most of the western diet tends to be based on refined grains. Another problem, according to Dr. Walter Willett, a Harvard nutritionist, is that the fat group has moved to the top, indicating to consume as little as possible, yet unsaturated fats, from a natural source, is essential in a person's general sustainability. The U.S.D.A. (United States Department of Agriculture), Food Pyramid recommends that carbohydrates should form sixty percent of your daily intake in calories. That actually converts to three hundred grams of sugar or almost eleven ounces of sugar daily! And we wonder why obesity is becoming epidemic!

Q:

Can you please explain the difference between food allergies and food intolerances and what are the common allergens?

A:

Food allergy and food intolerance are frequently lumped together as a single condition. However, in a true allergic reaction, the body releases histamine, which produces the gastrointestinal, respiratory, and skin symptoms associated allergies. Food intolerance can produce somewhat similar symptoms, but the chemistry is quite different-no histamine is released. Common causes of food intolerance include the absence of a digestive enzyme that is needed to digest a specific food fully, irritable bowel syndrome, stress and foods contaminated by toxins. One note to keep in mind is that if you have a food intolerance or food allergy it may not be the food itself but the substances or additives used in preparation of the food. The most common food reactions are lactose (usually from milk), gluten (found in wheat), MSG (monosodium glutamate) and food dyes & colorings.

Q:

I am taking a hypertensive medication and was told that I should not drink grapefruit juice. I started drinking pomegranate juice because of its health benefits but then I read that it interferes with absorption of the medication also. Is that correct? I really enjoy drinking the pomegranate juice.

A:

Continue your enjoyment! Because pomegranate juice has different properties than grapefruit juice, it has no effect on the absorption of any medications according to David J. Greenblatt, M.D., Professor of the Department of Pharmacology at Tuft's University. The problem with drinking grapefruit juice or eating grapefruit is that it inhibits a chemical in the intestine needed to break down the medication which results in an increased blood level of the medication. This caution of grapefruit also applies to certain cholesterol medications, so it is very important to consult with your physician or pharmacist about possible interactions. Just as a footnote, I would also recommend that you avoid Seville oranges as it interferes with the absorption of certain medications as well.

Q:

If I eat anything with MSG, I will develop a migraine headache. I am diligent in reading labels and try to avoid processed foods, but sometimes I will eat something that even though it does not list MSG on the label, I still get a migraine. Are there others names for MSG and if so, could you please list them.

A:

Monosodium Glutamate, MSG, is considered an excitotoxin and is an ingredient known to cause nerve damage by overexciting nerves, which is exactly how MSG enhances the taste of foods by overexciting the taste buds of the tongue. When you look at a food label, any of the following words indicate another name for MSG: Hydrolyzed vegetable protein, Maltodextrin, Textured protein, Sodium caseinate, Glutamic acid, Gelatin, Carrageenan (processed), Ultra-pasteurized, Pectin protease, Stock, Whey protein isolate, Whey protein, Barley malt, Malt extract, Natural Pork, Beef or Chicken flavoring, Citric acid (when processed from corn), Protease enzyme, Flavoring, Hydrolyzed yeast extract, Tortula yeast, Autolyzed yeast, Yeast extract, Soy protein, Pea protein, Wheat protein, Corn Protein, Soy protein concentrate, Textured soy protein, anything protein fortified , anything fermented and Dextrose. When any product contains seventy-nine percent free glutamic acid with the balance being made up of salt, moisture, and up to one percent contaminants, the product is called Monosodium Glutamate. If you are interested in learning more about the toxicity of MSG, *The Slow Poisoning of America* by John and Michelle Erb details studies that indicate that MSG is addictive (and MSG manufacturers openly admit it) and laboratory studies that MSG triples the amount of insulin the pancreas secretes resulting in obesity.

Q:

I am learning about the difference between Monounsaturated, Polyunsaturated and Saturated fat but was wondering if oils, like olive oil, contain all three, and if so, how much of each of these dietary fats are in different oils. I hope my question is clear.

A:

Dietary fats actually fall into four categories; Monounsaturated, Polyunsaturated, and Saturated fats that occur naturally in foods and the dreaded Trans Fats, that are man made fats, and should be avoided at all cost. All vegetable oils contain levels of Monounsaturated, Polyunsaturated and Saturated fats. Oils with a higher percentage of unsaturated fats are generally considered more healthful. Here is a sampling of oils and their different levels of fats. *Olive oil* is 72% Monounsaturated, 9% Polyunsaturated and 14% Saturated fat. *Flax oil* is 72% Monounsaturated, 19% Polyunsaturated and 9% Saturated fat. *Hempseed Oil* is 80% Monounsaturated, 12% Polyunsaturated and 8% Saturated fat. *Peanut Oil* is 46% Monounsaturated, 32% Polyunsaturated and 17% Saturated fat. *Corn Oil* is 24% Monounsaturated, 59% Polyunsaturated and 13% Saturated fat. *Coconut Oil* is 6% Monounsaturated, 2% Polyunsaturated, and 87% Saturated fat. *Sunflower Oil* is 20% Monounsaturated, 66% Polyunsaturated and 10% Saturated fat. A few facts to remember; dietary fat plays an important role in human health although we should not consume more than 10% of the daily diet in saturated fats. Also, dietary fats are carriers of fat soluble vitamins, are essential for energy, and are a source of essential fatty acids such as Omega 3 and Omega 6. Monounsaturated fats are found in avocados, nuts, seeds, olive oil and natural peanut butter. Polyunsaturated fats are found in fatty fish like salmon, walnuts, and sunflower seeds. Saturated fats are found in meat, diary and coconut oil. Trans fats are found in processed foods like hydrogenated margarine and foods fried in hydrogenated or partially hydrogenated vegetable oils like donuts or prepared with these hydrogenated oils like cookies, pastries, crackers and junk foods.

Q:

Can you please give me some information regarding digestive enzymes? Which ones are the most important and can overcooking vegetables cause a problem within the digestive system?

A:

Enzymes are a delicate substance found in all living cells whether animal or vegetable. Enzymes regulate and catalyze almost all biochemical reactions that occur in the human body. Our bodies naturally produce both digestive and metabolic enzymes. While the human body makes approximately twenty two digestive enzymes, there are four basic digestive enzymes; Protease-digests protein, Amylase digest non-fiber carbohydrates, Cellulase digest fiber and Lipase digests fats. Digestive enzymes are secreted along the digestive tract to break down food into nutrients and wastes. Metabolic enzymes speed up chemical reactions within the cells for detoxification and energy production. Overcooking vegetables not only destroys the natural plant enzymes, but it destroys the nutrients as well. Light heat on the cook top is acceptable, however, due to the commuting lifestyle of so many, the microwave is used and that kills all the enzymes and can leave the food toxic.

Q:

I have noticed that some diet sodas and juices say "Phenlyketonurics: Contains Phenylalanine". Can you please tell me what this is and why does this appear as a "warning"?

A:

Phenylalanine, which is an essential amino acid needed by the body, also happens to be a component of the artificial sweetener, Aspartame. Most individuals do not worry about the warning but phenylalanine can be a problem for those who suffer from a metabolic disorder called phenylketonuria or PKU. For individuals that are diagnosed with PKU, they lack an enzyme needed to process the amino acid, therefore consumption of phenylalanine can reach toxic levels in their blood and tissue. According to the Food and Drug Administration, it is required that any product with Aspartame must have this warning on the product label. Screening for PKU, now referred to as newborn screen, is now routine since mental retardation can result if a newborn's PKU goes undiagnosed.

Q:

Does the sodium in a natural food have less effect on blood pressure than the sodium found in processed foods?

A:

Sodium has the same effect on blood pressure, whether it is consumed as table salt, in processed foods or as it occurs naturally in foods. If you are monitoring your sodium intake, be diligent in totaling your sodium intake from all sources. Did you know that celery contains about 35 milligrams of sodium per stalk?

Q:

I have been taking a sustained-release form of niacin, but recently read that it can cause liver damage. Is taking the sustained release form more dangerous that the regular crystalline form? The crystalline form makes me flush.

A:

Research has indicated that both crystalline (short acting) and sustained-release (long acting) niacin can cause liver damage at high doses. However, as more research is being conducted, results indicate that the sustained-release form can cause liver damage even at low therapeutic doses. While the exact reason is unclear, the theory is that taking the short acting crystalline niacin allows the liver to recover between dosages, whereas the sustained-release niacin affects the liver enzymes for a longer period of time without a chance to recover. If you are a diabetic, I recommend that you DO NOT take any form of niacin since it can aggravate diabetes. Although niacin may be purchased over the counter, and I suggest the crystalline form in very low doses, be sure to consult with your physician before taking niacin or any supplements if you have been diagnosed with any medical disorder.

Q:

Can you give me any guidelines on when someone should take Probiotic supplements?

A:

Inside each of us live a vast number of bacteria, without which, we could not remain in good health. Of the several billion in each one of us, most live in the digestive tract. While some of the bacteria aid in maintaining good health, others help us regain health once it has been disrupted. The use of friendly bacteria supplements is known as probiotics. According to Deepak Chopra. M.D. here is a list of recommendations as to when you should use probiotics. 1) If there are chronic bowel problems or ongoing infections such as candidiasis. 2) As a preventive against food poisoning when traveling (Bifidobacteria and acidophilus kill most food poisoning bacteria). 3) After (and during) any antibiotic use. 4) By all premenopausal and menopausal women to reduce chances of osteoporosis. 5) By anyone with high cholesterol problems. 6) By anyone with chronic health problems (acne, skin problems, allergies, arthritis, cancer). 7) By anyone receiving radiation treatment. 8) By anyone having recurrent vaginal or bladder infections (thrush or cystitis) and as a footnote, Bifidobacteria infantis should be given to all babies. As I always suggest, consult with your physician and inform him/her of all supplements that you are taking including probiotics, and read the labels. Avoid purchasing probiotic supplements that are synthetic or that contain synthetic additives like maltodextrin.

Q:

Can you please explain the difference between soluble fiber and insoluble fiber? Is one more important than the other?

A:

Insoluble fiber is not soluble in water as the name suggests (unlike soluble fiber). Insoluble fiber is often referred to as roughage since it aids in moving bulk through the intestines, helps control and balance the pH (potential of hydrogen or acidity) in the intestines, promotes regular bowel movements and removes toxic waster through the colon is less time. Food sources of insoluble fiber are vegetables, dark green leafy vegetables, fruit skins, root vegetable skins, bran, whole grains, seeds and nuts. Soluble fiber, on the other hand, helps carry cholesterol out of the body in bile, and slows the rate at which the stomach empties (so that sugar is released and absorbed more slowly). Food sources of soluble fiber are oat/oat bran, dried beans and peas, nuts, barley, flax seeds, oranges, apples, bananas, berries, pears, sweet potatoes, broccoli, and carrots. While soluble fiber and insoluble fiber differ significantly, each of them have an important role in the development and nourishment of the body and one should include a blend of both types of fiber in their diet.

Q:

This past week I was diagnosed with drug induced Lupus. My physician took me off of the suspect medication and the symptoms are beginning to subside. Can you tell what I need to change and about a diet that can help the rash and other symptoms I developed go away a bit faster?

A:

Drug-induced lupus erythematosus (DILE) is caused by a reaction with certain prescription drugs and can cause symptoms very similar to systemic lupus erythematosus (SLE) which is an autoimmune disease. If you smoke, it is critical to stop smoking. Stay out of the sun as much as possible, an unfortunate recommendation since you need Vitamin D and twenty minutes in the sun every day is the best source. Therefore, you might want to consider taking a Vitamin D supplement. It is important to get enough sleep, during the night, not just "cat naps" during the day. Sleeping during night allows the body to regenerate and helps cleanse the liver and kidneys. Your diet is by far the most important change you can make. Limiting or better yet, avoiding sugar, even artificial sweeteners, is most beneficial as well as eliminating caffeine. Limiting salt intake is important if you are on corticosteroids. Some research indicates that eating more fish (not farm raised) can be beneficial since it has anti-inflammatory properties. Avoid alfalfa sprouts since they may increase inflammation. Drinking plenty of water benefits the systems by flushing out toxins, so my recommendation of drinking half of your body weight in ounces of water daily can be a key factor. For more information you can contact the Lupus Foundation of America, 2000 L Street, N.W.

Suite 710, Washington, DC 20036 or you can visit their web site, www.lupus.org.

Q:

Since this is the cold season, I would like to know your thoughts on taking zinc lozenges. Does it really help if you have a cold to take zinc lozenges?

A:

Zinc is an essential mineral that is found is almost every cell. Zinc supports normal immune function, interferes with viral replication, and is important for tissue repair. Zinc can decrease the ability of the cold virus to grow on or bind to the nasal lining of the nose according to web.md. The real secret to taking zinc lozenges is to take it at the first symptoms of a cold, every two hours, because not taking zinc with regularity during the initial stages of the cold reduces its effectiveness dramatically. It is important to remember, however, that you should not take zinc for longer than five days at a time and zinc IS NOT recommended for children. Tea, coffee and certain medications may interfere with zinc absorption in the intestines. If you must have a hot cup of tea or coffee, naturally decaffeinated is recommended. When selecting a zinc lozenge, be sure to read the label. A little added Vitamin C is great but you will not benefit from a lozenge with a lot of additives.

Q:

You have mentioned in your column about avoiding Genetically Modified Organisms. As I read more labels, I do find more products that state that it DOES NOT contain GMO's, although I have never seen a label that says it DOES contain GMO's. So, my questions are: Does the FDA (Food and Drug Administration) regulate GMO's found in food? When did they come about? Can you please explain exactly what GMO's are, one more time?

A:

The simple answer to your first question: NO. Genetically Modified Organisms (GMO's) do not require approval by the FDA prior to availability at your local markets. The FDA puts responsibility on the company developing the food for its safety. Since GMO's in foods were only introduced in 1994, there have been no long term studies on the safety of eating genetically modified foods and therefore the long term health effects are unknown. GMO's refer to crop plants created for human or animal consumption using the latest bio-technology. These products are genetically engineered so that they are more pest resistant (to lower crop cost from insect damage), herbicide tolerant (too costly to pick the weeds), disease resistant (engineered to resists viruses, fungi and bacteria that can disease a plant), cold tolerant (unexpected frost can destroy seedlings), and drought tolerant (planting crops in unfavorable locations). This altering process has left about sixty five percent of the food on the grocery shelves containing genetically modified ingredients. An example, more than eighty percent of cheese is produced using a genetically engineered enzyme known as chymosin. More and more food manufacturers are indicating if their product is NON-GMO by wording or by a red circle with the slash through GMO. Keep reading your food labels!

Q:

I have been diagnosed with heart disease and told I have an elevated homocysteine level. How do you reduce homocysteine levels in your system through nutrition?

A:

Homocysteine, is an amino acid in the blood. There are two factors to the problem of a high homocysteine level. One is the amount of methionine, also an amino acid, in your diet that the body has to metabolize and break down. It is important to add enough fruits and vegetables and carefully moniter the amount of foods that are high in saturated fats like meat and dairy. The second factor is providing enough folic acid, and vitamins B6 and B12 so that the enzyme systems needed to break down homocysteine can work effectively. Foods high in folic acid include green, leafy vegetables and gluten free grain products fortified with folic acid. According to the American Heart Association, homocysteine levels are strongly influenced by diet. Because our food is so over processed, I recommend fresh vegetables rather than canned vegetables (remember they are cooked in the can), and fresh fruits.

Q:

I have been desperately trying to loose weight but find myself struggling every day. I am making healthier choices in my food and have changed my lifestyle in that I am eating more regularly, but admit I do not always eat breakfast. I do drink a few diet sodas a day-they are not that bad are they? Quite often, by the end of the day I have wilted. What else can I change? I appreciate your help.

A:

Congrats to you for realizing how important a good weight is and how critical the role a healthy diet plays. One of the most important factors in a healthy lifestyle is to always begin your day by eating breakfast. I am not talking about a seven course buffet style breakfast but something as simple and easy as a good health bar, simply because something is much better than nothing and of course, WATER. If you choose to have a bit more for breakfast, a bowl of one hundred percent rolled oats, cream of wheat or other healthy choices make for a better start. Your body has regenerated all night during your sleep (I hope you are sleeping all thru the night?) and is ready for some replenishment upon awakening, which is actually why we call it breakfast (we break the fast). Also, if you take a whole food multi vitamin it is important that you take it with food, and breakfast is a great meal to get you going for the day. About the sodas-even though they are one hundred percent calorie free, they are also one hundred percent nutrition free. And if you are drinking the soda out of an aluminum can, that is beginning the day with toxins. Have you ever noticed a plant that has wilted? Usually the first thing you do is to pour WATER on the plant, not a diet soda, or coffee or anything else, just water. Within a short time, the plant has perked back up! Our bodies respond the same way, so I would suggest you try and drink more WATER, especially with your breakfast and even better if you can continue throughout the day. Did you know that your BRAIN is about 70% water, your MUSCLE is about 75% water, your BONE is about 97% water, your BODY FAT is about ½% water, your LUNGS are about 90% water, and your BLOOD is about 80% water? Remember, you need to drink one half of your body weight in ounces of water daily. That is, if you weight one hundred and sixty pounds, you will need to drink eighty ounces of water daily. That old adage "watch what you eat" is just as important as "watch what you drink". And remember, both are just as important as to the quantity! Let's not wilt!

Q:

For years I have eaten garlic and taken garlic tablets because I have always heard how beneficial garlic is to the system. I hope what I have always heard is correct but I do wonder what exactly is in garlic that makes it so healthy? I hope what I have been doing for years is on track!

A:

You are right on track! Allicin is the mystery compound found in garlic that has antibacterial, antifungal, and antimicrobial effects. Although allicin (al-e-sin) was only discovered in 1944 by an Italian chemist, C. J. Cavallito, ancient cultures around the world had all come to the same conclusion about the ability of garlic to fight disease. Allicin is produced by the garlic plant as a defense against pests but once inside your body, allicin becomes the body's best defense mechanism. Allicin does not occur in "ordinary" garlic, but is actually activated once you crush the garlic or chop it as finely as possible. The finer the garlic is chopped or crushed, the more allicin is generated, and the stronger the medicinal effect. To achieve the most benefit of the allicin, it is best to add the crushed or chopped garlic to a food just prior to serving since it degrades quickly after it has been produced. Microwaving destroys all of the benefits of allicin immediately (one more reason NOT TO MICROWAVE).

Q:

Can you please settle an argument? Is turkey bacon better than pork bacon?

A:

In several surveys that I have conducted, just asking individuals which is they think is healthier, turkey bacon or pork bacon, turkey bacon always wins! But the truth is Pork is the best and for several reasons. First off, most turkey bacon has a laundry list of ingredients indicating too many processed additives, 2) some brands include soy, 3) most include some form of sweetener (i.e., sugar, dextrose or maltodextrin), and 4) most turkey bacon contains more sodium and cholesterol. While the turkey bacon does contain a leaner source of meat, it is not one hundred percent turkey, hence all of the additives. It is very important to read the labels even though the nutritional statement on the front of the package does not always mean it is healthy. As an example, some brands of turkey bacon state on the front of the package that it is 50% less fat, which is usually a red flag indicating something else has been added to compensate for the difference. Buyer Beware!

Q:

I am writing this letter since I am too old to learn how to do a computer. I love raspberry candy and have eaten it for many years as a treat. Since reading your articles, I look at the label more. The candy I bought says it has castoreum in it. What is castoreum? I know what the others ingredients are.

A:

I hope you still enjoy your candy after I tell you what castoreum is. Castoreum is actually beaver anal glands and is used to enhance the flavor of raspberry candies. It is also uses in perfumes, cigarettes and if you are thinking about changing to chewing gum-well, castoreum is also in some chewing gums!

Q:

Over the past year I have been drinking green tea, that is decaffeinated, and I really enjoy it. However, I wonder if there is any other tea, that has as many health benefits, is decaffeinated, and one that has some flavor since the green tea is a bit limited on flavor?

A:

Your choice of tea is good since there are so many to choose from; Black, Oolong, White, Green, Chai, Flavored, Blended, Herbal, and Blooms, but the one I would recommend, hands down for the best flavor and one that is all natural is Rooibos Tea. Because I always say if you cannot pronounce it-do not consume it, I will tell you the proper pronunciation is ROY-bose. When I say this tea is all natural, it contains very little oxalic acid (so it good for individuals with kidney disorders), and has low tannin levels so it is easier for people to drink with acid reflux. In addition, Rooibos is high in polyphenols, and contain no colors, no additives, no preservatives and best of all-no caffeine. Rooibos tea is an excellent thirst quencher, great for athletes and active individuals including children since it is naturally decaffeinated. This tea, grows only near the Cape of Good Hope in South Africa, and has been researched by scientist Dr. Jeanie Marnewick, in clinical trials and the results indicated that Rooibos tea is beneficial in individuals with insomnia, irritability, headaches, nervous tension and hypertension. If you prefer a sweeter flavor, you can drizzle a bit of honey or agave nectar into your Rooibos to enhance the excellent flavor.

Q:

I read so many health claims on packaging that I am totally confused. How much of this stuff is true? Some products claim if you eat certain foods, you can reduce your risk of cancer. I am a cancer survivor and want to be sure I am eating the right foods but it is difficult since so many foods are processed and genetically modified. Is there a list of claims that are credible?

A:

There are abundant health claims, but there are only twelve health claims linking the use of a food to a reduced risk of a specific disease that have been approved by the Food and Drug Administration. Here is the list: Calcium rich foods *and* reduced risk of osteoporosis, Low Sodium foods *and* reduced risk of high blood pressure, Low Fat diet *and* reduced risk of cancer, A diet low in saturated fat and cholesterol *and* reduced risk of heart disease, High fiber foods *and* reduced risk of cancer, Soluble fiber in fruits, vegetables, and grains *and* reduced risk of heart disease, Soluble Fiber in oats and psyllium seed husk *and* reduced risk of heart disease, Fruit and Vegetable rich diet *and* reduced risk of cancer, Folate rich foods *and* reduced risk of neural tube defects, Less sugar *and* reduced risk of dental caries, Monounsaturated fat from olive oil *and* reduced risk of coronary heart disease and Tree nuts *and* the reduced risk for heart disease.

Q:

In terms of potential health benefits, is it better to consume whole flaxseeds or flaxseed oil?

A:

Flaxseeds are the better choice. Flaxseed oil, unlike plain flaxseed, does not contain lignans-plant estrogens that are believed to protect against breast, prostate and other hormone-sensitive cancers according to Tufts University. The oil also lacks soluble fiber, the type of oil associated with lower blood cholesterol. In addition, flaxseed oil has poor stability, with an optimum shelf life-even in the refrigerator-of only six weeks. And, flaxseed oil is not as widely available as flaxseeds, which are now available in most supermarkets. An important note to remember is that in order for the health benefits of the flaxseeds to be attainable, the seeds must be ground. If not, they simply pass through the gastrointestinal tract whole and can cause problems if you suffer from diverticulosis or diverticulitis.

Q:

I absolutely love to eat black pepper-I put it on everything! Can you share with me a little history about black pepper? Does pepper have any nutrient value?

A:

Pepper comes from the seed or fruit of a shrub which originally grew on the western coast of India. Today it is grown and cultivated in Malaysia, China, Sri Lanka, Madagascar, and South America with eighty percent coming from Indonesia. While black pepper can grow wild, most of it is cultivated on plantations. The pepper plants require constant trimming and fertilization and the underbrush must be constantly cut away. The pepper berry is green at first, then turns yellow and is picked when it turns red just before it is quite ripe. This is because they are more pungent at this time. They are then spread out to dry in the sun. After they are dried-they turn black. White pepper is not as strong and is made from ripe berries from which the outer coat has been removed before grinding. A pepper shrub will yield fruit in three years and will reach full production by the time the plant is seven years old.

Peppercorns are very rich in vitamin A and K, is a good source of dietary fiber and contains calcium, magnesium, potassium, manganese, phosphorous and beta carotene.

Q:

Some time back you listed some food trivia facts and since I understand you like trivia, I am just wondering if you would consider listing some more facts? Thanks for your consideration!

A:

I do love trivia, so here are a few trivia facts you might find interesting. Worcestershire sauce is made from dissolved anchovies. The most expensive coffee in the world comes from civet poop. Coca-cola would be green if coloring was not added to it. On average, a pound of potato chips cost two hundred times more than a pound of potatoes. Only five out of one hundred pounds of salt ends up on the dinner table-the rest is used for such diverse purposes as packing meat, building roads, feeding livestock, tanning leather, and manufacturing glass, soap, ash, and washing compounds. There are fifteen thousand different kinds of rice. Refined sugar is the only food known to provide calories but has no nutritional value. After the "Popeye" comic strip started in the 1930's, spinach consumption went up by thirty three percent in the United States. It takes food seven seconds to get from your mouth to your stomach.

Q:

I was recently diagnosed with cancer and was told that my system was acidic. I have since read that your pH must be balanced in order for your system to be healthy. My questions for you are: Can you please explain what pH is? Is there a general rule on what foods are acidic or alkaline? And, is there any suggested reading regarding pH balance that you could recommend?

A:

The acid/alkaline balance of your system is referred to as pH, which is an acronym for potential of hydrogen. Without going into the chemistry detail, the most important factor to remember is that ideal pH is neutral at 7.0. A pH below 7.0 is considered acid while a reading above 7.0 is considered alkaline. It is critical that the body stay balanced at 7.0. Because so much of the Western diet contains highly processed and genetically modified foods, its can cause an imbalance in the blood pH which can lead to irritation and inflammation and sets the stage for sickness. (The movie Supersize Me is a prime example). Having lived abroad for almost twenty years observing diets and lifestyles, those countries where individuals consumed diets of live food rather than over processed foods, their pH maintained balance and therefore their health was exceptional. Foods are classified as acid forming (meats, processed food, dairy) or alkalizing (vegetables, most citrus fruits, nuts) depending on the effect they have on the body, therefore, it is important to eat eighty percent alkaline foods and twenty percent acid forming foods. For a short list of acid/alkaline foods, you can visit my web site, www.docphyl.com, and I highly recommend reading *The pH Miracle* by Robert O. Young, Ph.D.

Q:

Since reading your weekly column, I have become more aware of food labels and am trying to get in the habit of reading them. I happened to read the food label on a container of No Sugar Added light ice cream that I have had in the freezer and noticed one of the ingredients was Acesulfame Potassium. I know you say if you cannot pronounce the ingredient, you should not eat it. Now that I am almost done with it, I am sure if you can explain to me what it is I will not buy another!

A:

Acesulfame Potassium , acesulfame-K, or ACK, is a calorie free, artificial sweetener that is frequently used with other artificial sweeteners to mask bitterness. The Food and Drug Administration approved ACK almost fifteen years ago but according to David Zincenko, author of Eat This Not That, some health groups claimed the decision was based on flawed tests. Animal studies have linked ACK to lung and breast tumors. Based on my research, and according to the Department of Environmental and Occupational Health, further studies have been requested on the safety of ACK. As a footnote, I could tell you how to pronounce acesulfame but if I did, I would not be benefiting you- I can tell you to avoid products that contain this ingredient.

Index

CPSIA information can be obtained at www.ICGtesting.com
Printed in the USA
LVOW05s0539160813

348119LV00003B/261/P